FAMILY MEDICAL HANDBOOK

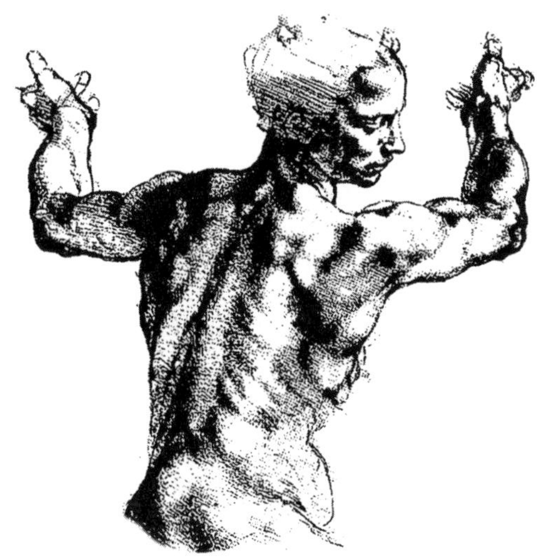

YOUR HOME GUIDE TO HEALTH AND BASIC EMERGENCY CARE

Mervyn G. Hardinge, M.D., Dr. P.H., Ph.D.
Harold Shryock, M.A., M.D.
In collaboration with 28 leading medical specialists

Pacific Press® Publishing Association
Nampa, ID 83653
Oshawa, Ontario, Canada

Photo and illustration credits:
Pages 39, 40 Lucille Innes.
Pages 19, 20, 22, 24 Duane Tank.
Page 27 Duane Tank/Betty Blue.

Please Note: Although the information contained in the *Family Medical Handbook* is based on accurate, reliable medical knowledge, it is designed to be of a general nature and for informational purposes only. The *Family Medical Handbook* is not intended to be used for self-diagnosis of medical problems nor to determine treatment apart from your physician. The publishers are not responsible for your decisions based on your use of the content of the *Family Medical Handbook*. Always consult your physician when medical attention is indicated.

Edited by Marvin Moore/Bonnie Tyson-Flyn
Cover photo—Mark Vandersys
Cover design—Dennis Ferree
Design and art direction—Robert N. Mason, Flying Moose Designs
Art and illustration direction—Lars Justinen, Justinen Creative Group Inc.
Illustrators—Randy Jamison, Lars Justinen, Kevin McCain, Dan Pape
Line illustrations—Kim Justinen

ISBN 0-8163-1791-7

00 01 02 03 04 • 6 5 4 3 2 1

CONTENTS

Important emergency procedures

Chapter Outline

- Artificial respiration
- Cardiopulmonary resuscitation
- Initiating vomiting
- Combating shock
- Dressings and bandages
- Bleeding

Learn them before you need them

The basic support systems of the body are circulation and respiration, for without these functions, life cannot be sustained. To effectively support these systems, **Basic Life Support** (**BLS**) procedures have been designed to intervene when these systems are assessed to need intervention. Indications for **BLS** are:

- **Primary respiratory arrest.** The heart is able to circulate the blood until all of the oxygen present in the blood and lungs has been depleted, at which time the vital organs, such as the brain and heart, will cease to function, and the heart will stop beating (cardiac arrest). A person will stop breathing (respiratory arrest) from a number of causes. These include drowning, an object in the airway, suffocation, smoke inhalation, stroke, drug overdose, heart attack, injuries, and coma.
- **Primary cardiac arrest.** When the heart stops beating, blood is not circulated, and the oxygen in the blood is used up by the tissues and organs in a matter of seconds. Among the causes for the heart to stop beating are a massive heart attack, fibrillation (twitching) of the ventricles, and beating too fast (tachycardia).

The major important emergency procedures that are needed from time to time in rendering first aid to someone who is injured or seriously ill are outlined below. They are called the ABCs of cardiopulmonary resuscitation (CPR).

1. Airway—see that it is open.
2. Breathing—give artificial respiration.
3. Circulation—provide external chest compression.

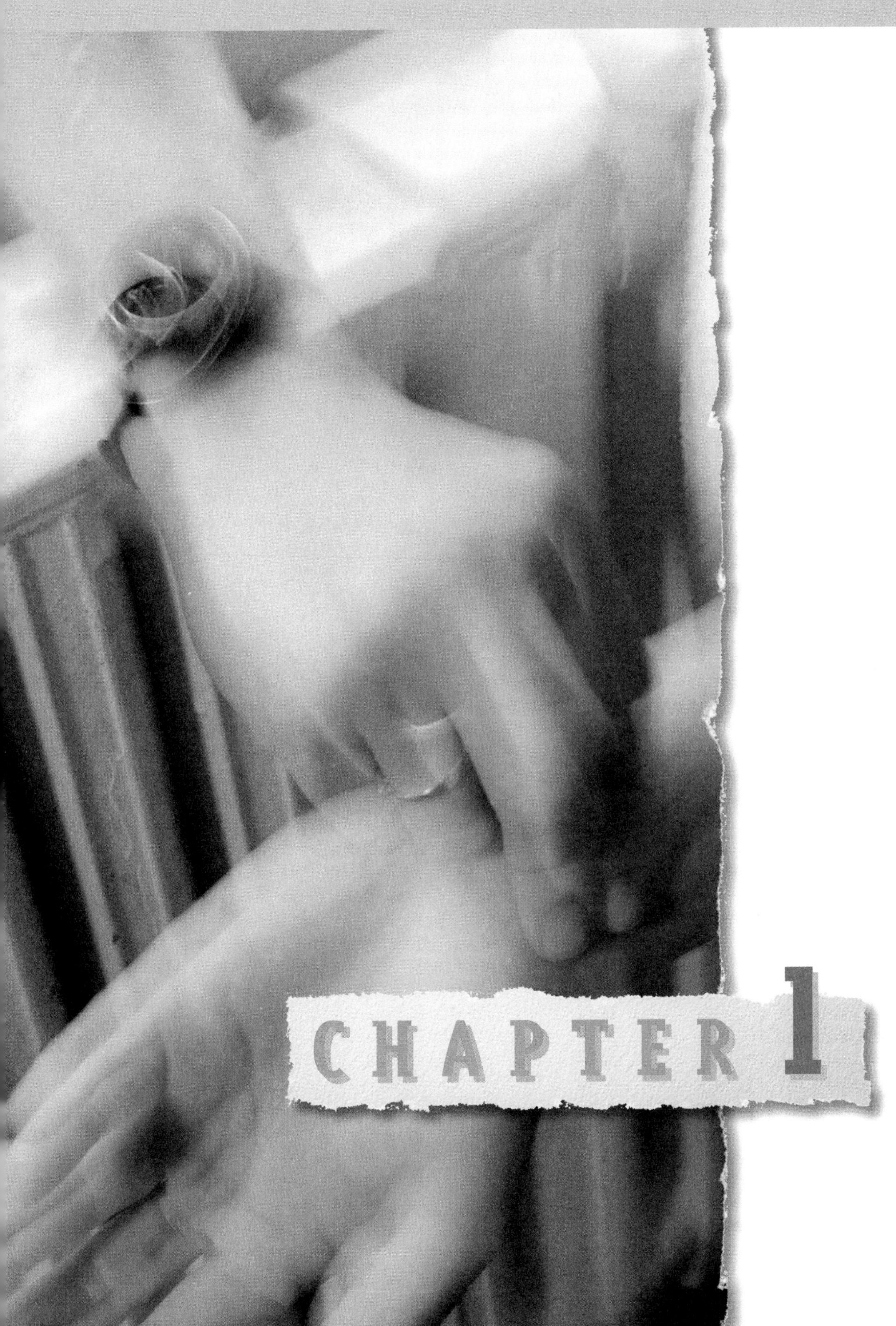

CHAPTER 1

Artificial respiration

Artificial respiration can be given even if breathing has not entirely stopped, but is very slow and weak. Time your breathing **out** with the victim's breathing **in**.

Step 1

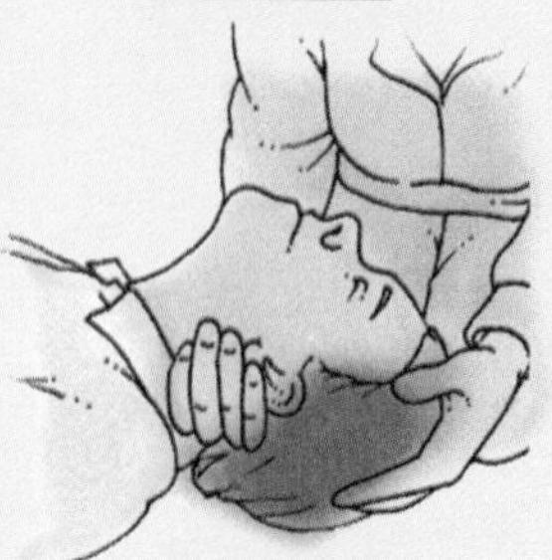

A. Lay the victim on his back.
B. Establish unresponsiveness. Is the victim unconscious?
C. Look for chest movement, and place your ear to his mouth to check for breathing.
D. Call for help.

Step 2

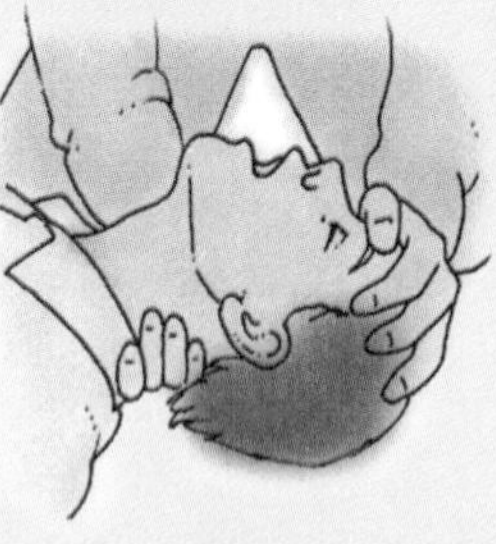

"Chin lift," *if no neck injury is suspected.*

A. Tilt the victim's head to a "sniffing" position (as when you smell a rose) by lifting up his neck with one hand while pushing back on his forehead with the other.
B. Pinch the victim's tongue and chin between your fingers. Wipe any foreign material from his mouth (using your finger and a handkerchief), and see that his tongue has not fallen backward.

Step 3

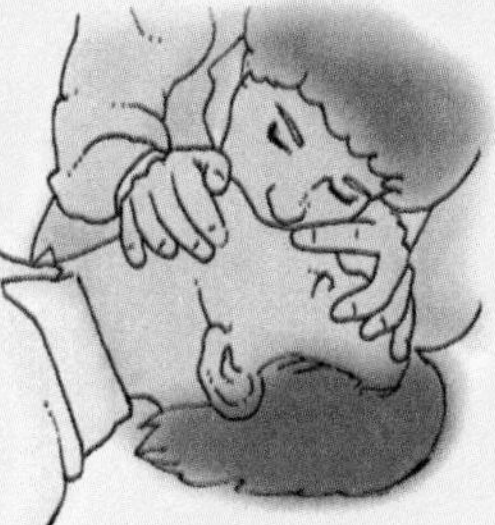

Pinch the victim's nose shut, take a deep breath, place your mouth firmly over his mouth, and give two quick breaths in rapid succession. In children cover both nose and mouth with your mouth.

Step 4

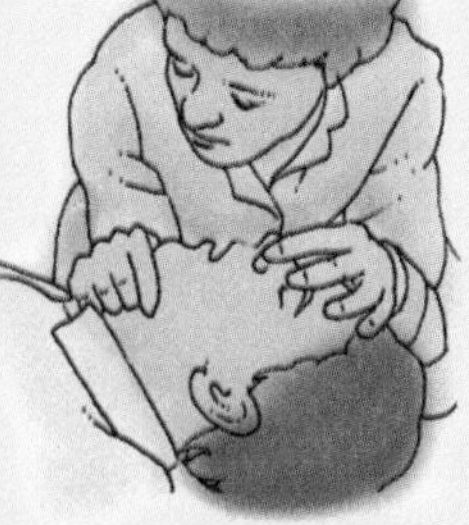

Remove your mouth from the victim's face. **Look** toward his chest so you can observe it fall, and **listen** to the sound of escaping air. **Feel** his breath on your face. If you feel none, try exhaling into his mouth again, more vigorously this time. If his chest still does not rise, the windpipe is obstructed. If the victim is a child, slap sharply between the shoulders and clear the mouth of any obstructing material. If the victim is an adult, use the Heimlich maneuver (see page 48).

Step 5

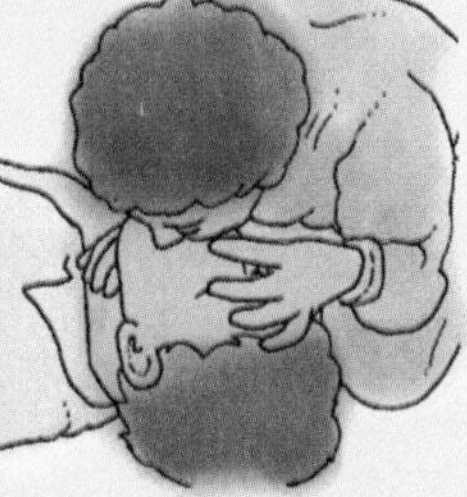

Continue blowing air into the victim's lungs every five seconds (twelve to fourteen times a minute) until he resumes normal breathing or until help arrives.

Caution: When giving mouth-to-mouth respiration to infants or very small children, ***remember*** *that their lung capacity is small.* ***Do not overinflate a child's lungs.*** *Only empty the air you can hold in your cheeks. Give gentle, small exhalations and watch the child's chest rise and fall. If the airway is obstructed, hold the child by the feet and gently thump between the shoulder blades.*

Cardiopulmonary resuscitation

When the heart stops beating, the circulation of blood ceases, and soon thereafter breathing terminates. An emergency measure called cardiopulmonary resuscitation (CPR) has saved many lives and is now well established. Everyone should avail himself of the first opportunity to learn from qualified teachers how to conduct this procedure. Many hospitals, fire departments, and the American Red Cross have training programs for the public in CPR An outline of the procedure is given below, but does not attempt to provide sufficient details to make the reader an efficient CPR operator.

When two rescuers are available, one can administer artificial respiration while the other carries out heart resuscitation. However, there may be only one rescuer who knows the procedure. **Laypersons should do single-rescue technique only.**

Step 1

Establish the victim's unresponsiveness—that he is unconscious: look, listen, feel.

Step 2

Call for help.

Step 3 Lay the victim on his back on a firm surface, such as on the floor. His arms should be parallel to his sides, and his head should be slightly lower than his chest. **Note: If there is a possible neck injury, avoid moving the victim's neck as you position him.**

Step 4 Tilt the victim's head back, and with one hand behind his neck, raise it upward. This will bring his chin up and open his airway. Clear his mouth of any foreign materials. The ideal head-neck position is "sniffing" (as if smelling a rose).

Step 5 Give two quick breaths.

Step 6 Check the victim's pulse.

Step 7 In adults, place a finger in the notch at the lower end of the victim's breastbone. Place the base of one of your palms 1 inch (2.5 cm) above the finger in the notch. Now remove the finger from the notch and place that hand on the back of the other hand. Keep your arms straight while kneeling at right angles to the victim.

Step 8 Push straight down, compressing the chest of an **adult** 1-1/2 to 2 inches (4 cm), smoothly and regularly. Between compressions, keep your hands lightly in contact with his chest (so your fingers are raised off the skin). Give eighty compressions per minute. Your timing will be "one-and," "two-and," "three-and"-slightly faster than one per second.

Step 9 **After fifteen compressions, lean forward, tip the victim's head, and give him two full breaths in four seconds.**

Step 10 After every minute or two, check the victim's pulse (preferably in the neck) and breathing for five seconds. **Look** for the rise of the chest, **listen** to breath sounds, and **feel** his breath on your face. Start each cycle with two breaths.

Evaluation. If on checking you find that the victim is breathing and has a good pulse, keep checking both periodically, and call for help. If you find only a pulse, then give mouth-to-mouth respiration. If you find no pulse, then start CPR. Continue CPR until help arrives or until you are exhausted. If the victim must be moved, do not stop CPR for more than fifteen seconds.

Caution. *For infants and small children, the force of compression should not bruise the heart or fracture the ribs. In babies, the pressure should be gentle, exerted through the tips of the operator's index and long fingers. In eight- to ten-year-olds, apply pressure with the heel of one hand.*

Cardiopulmonary resuscitation (CPR) in infants and small children. Note the location of the notch just below the breast bone and how the rescuer applies pressure to the chest using only his second and third fingers.

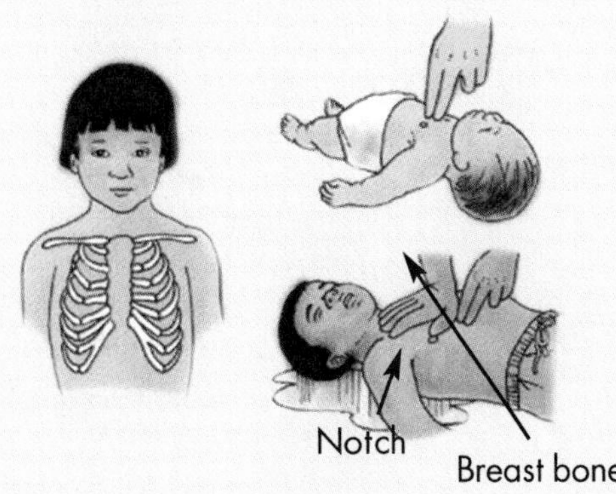

Before instituting any emergency procedure, there must be an assessment of the victim. The assessment involves:
1
Response—Is the victim conscious?
2
Breath—Is the victim breathing?
3
Pulse—Is the victim's heart beating?

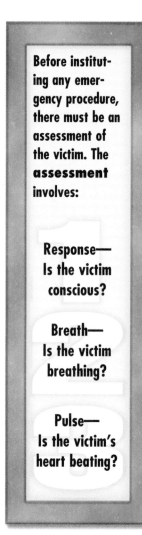

Initiating vomiting

Vomiting is a way of ridding the stomach of poisonous contents (if induced within thirty minutes).

Caution. Vomiting is not advised if the individual is unconscious or has swallowed a strong acid, a strong alkali, or a petroleum product.

Step 1 If necessary, position the victim so that the vomitus will flow out of his mouth and not be inhaled.

Step 2 Give the victim syrup of ipecac: 1 tablespoonful for children; 2 tablespoonfuls for adults. Follow this with two or more glasses of water or milk. If vomiting does not occur within fifteen minutes, tickle the back of the victim's throat with your finger or with the blunt end of a spoon, fork, or knife.

Combating shock

Shock can result from any number of causes, including a heart attack, severe injuries, acute infections, poisonings, hemorrhage, allergic responses, snakebites, and burns. In shock, there is a sudden collapse of the circulatory system, preventing the body's vital organs (the brain, kidneys, and the heart and blood vessels themselves) from receiving oxygen. If this situation is not corrected immediately, the spiral of failing function continues downward until it becomes irreversible. Following are three major causes of shock and what to do about them:

The heart fails to pump sufficient blood, as may occur in an acute coronary attack, heart failure, or cardiac arrest (**cardiogenic shock**).

There is insufficient blood in the arteries and veins, making it impossible for the body to maintain blood pressure. This may result from injuries, severe bleeding, burns, and diarrhea (**traumatic or hypovolemic shock**).

The blood vessels collapse, which causes them to dilate unduly. The blood pools, and there is insufficient blood to maintain circulation. This condition is usually seen in severe infections and in severe allergic reactions (**anaphylactic or distributive shock**).

The common symptoms of shock include generalized weakness; sweating; clammy skin; weak pulse; rapid, shallow breathing; and restlessness. As shock worsens there are mental haziness, lethargy, stupor, and unconsciousness. The victim's body temperature drops, and death ensues.

Dressings and bandages

Emergencies frequently involve injuries of the skin and bones. A **dressing** (also called a **compress**), usually composed of a fabric, is applied directly over the wound. While sterile (germ-free) dressings are commercially available, in an emergency, any cloth, or even paper, will do, provided it is relatively clean. Even tissues can be used.

The purpose of a dressing is to control bleeding, prevent further contamination, absorb blood or secretions, and prevent pain.

A **bandage** is a strip of cloth or woven material wrapped around a dressing to hold it in place. Bandages are also used with splints to prevent movement. Adhesive bandages are common examples of a combination dressing and bandage. Sterile gauze bandages of different widths are used to exert firm pressure on underlying tissues, helping to control bleeding.

A bandage should be snug, but not so tight that it will restrict the circulation of blood. After applying a bandage to a limb or finger, check to see that the area beyond the bandage is warm, and, when possible, check the pulse. As an injury swells, a bandage may become too tight and should be loosened.

A bandage must be held in place. A bandage that wraps around a limb or the head can be held in place with safety pins or clips, or, if it is a cloth bandage, it can be split and tied. A bandage can also be affixed directly to the skin with adhesive tape.

Bandages come in a variety of shapes and sizes and must be skillfully applied to conform to the

Treating shock

1 **Step 1:** Check the victim's circulation and respiration and, if needed, provide life-support procedures. Control any bleeding.

2 **Step 2:** Lay the victim down, and if other conditions (injuries) permit, raise his feet and legs about 1 foot (30 cm).

3 **Step 3:** Keep the victim warm to prevent loss of body heat.

4 **Step 4:** Call for medical help or take the victim to an emergency room.

5 **Step 5:** If the victim can cooperate, encourage him to drink water (unless he is vomiting), or, if it is available, a salt-soda solution (salt, 1 teaspoonful [4 gm]; soda, 1/2 teaspoonful [2 gm] to 1 quart [1 liter] of water).

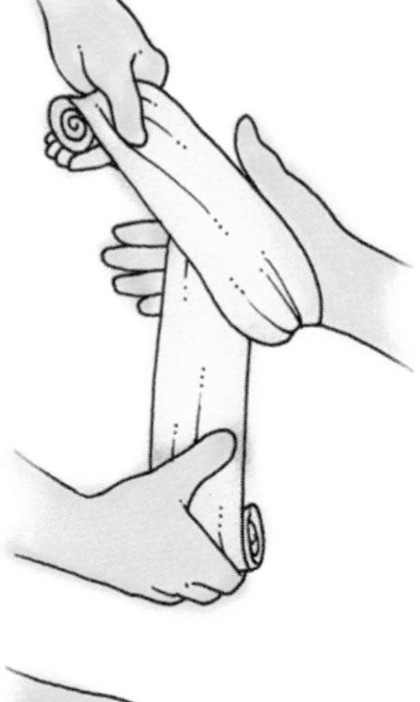

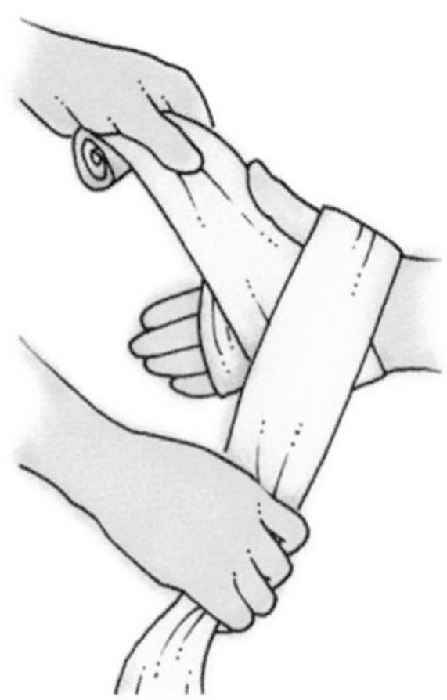

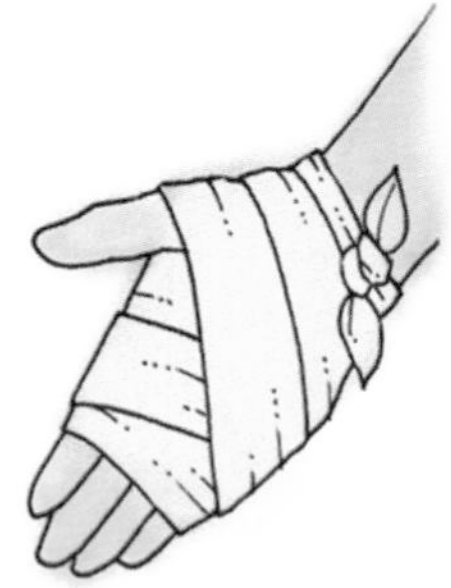

Application of a bandage to the hand.

varying contours of different parts of the head, body, and limbs. Common bandages include the sterile gauze roller bandage, the roller elastic bandage, and the triangular bandage (which may be a square folded in half). The stretch in the roller gauze bandage and the elastic bandage allows a snug fit around the varying shapes of the limbs. A triangular bandage can be used as a sling for suspending a limb (see the accompanying illustrations).

Bandaging is a learned skill. The reader is advised to obtain a booklet, the American Red Cross's *Standard First Aid*, and practice bandaging various parts of the body with different bandages. You will then be better prepared to meet an emergency.

Bleeding

Excessive bleeding (hemorrhaging), both internal and external, are life-threatening problems that require immediate attention to prevent death. Internal bleeding requires professional medical attention, and all you will be able to do is watch and give first aid for shock (see page 10). There are several ways to stop the flow of external blood loss, depending on the nature of the injury and where it is located. With the exception of the tourniquet, which is discussed below, the details of how to control bleeding are found on pages 44, 45.

A tourniquet is rarely if ever necessary, since direct pressure over the artery proximal to the point of bleeding (nearer the heart) should control the flow of blood. If applied, the condition should be a **life-threatening hemorrhage**, since limbs that are deprived of blood may require amputation. The material required is a wide bandage 2 to 4 inches wide (5 to 10 cm) or cloth torn from a sheet that is folded so it is several layers thick. Wrap the cloth around the bleeding arm or leg twice, just above the bleeding wound, and tie it with an overhand knot. Place a strong, short stick or similar article on the knot, and tie two additional knots on top of the stick. Now twist the stick so that it tightens the tourniquet. It is best to remove a tourniquet only on the advice of a physician.

Write a note indicating the location of the tourniquet and the time it was applied. This note can be written on the victim's forehead or on any writing material that is visible. Use an indelible pen, a pencil, or even lipstick.

Every family should have immediately available a first-aid book published by the American Red Cross. This book describes

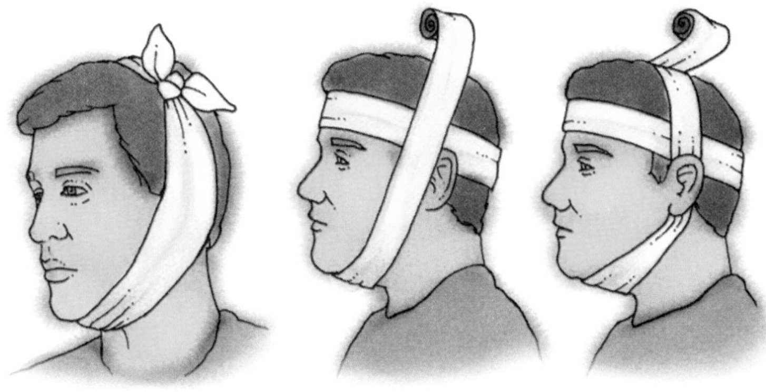

Scalp/head bandaging

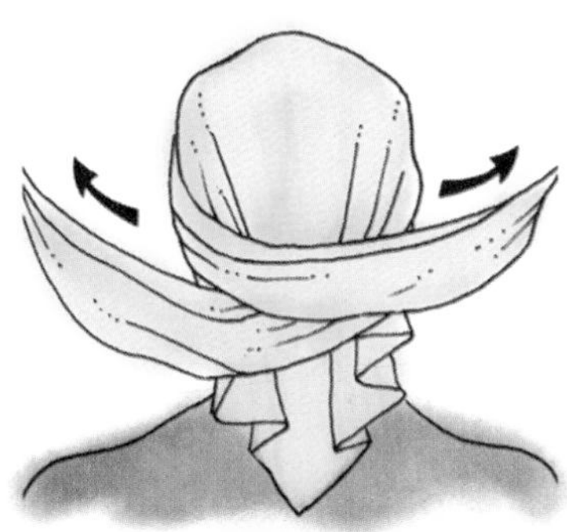

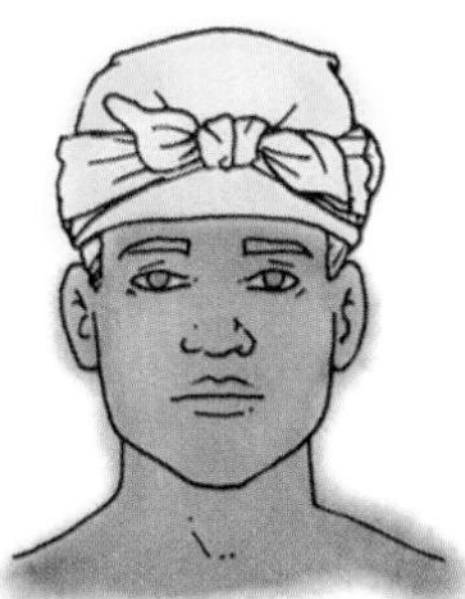

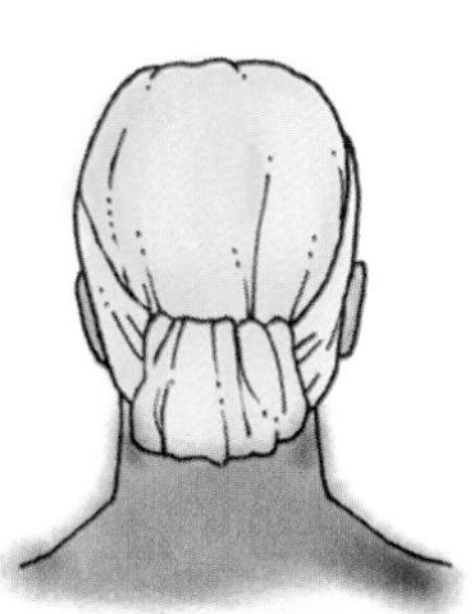

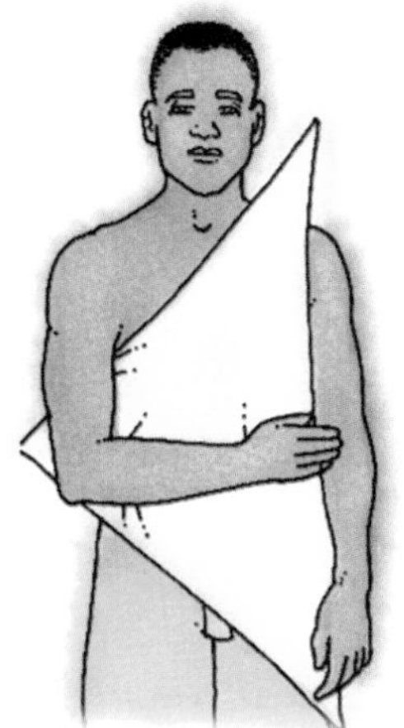

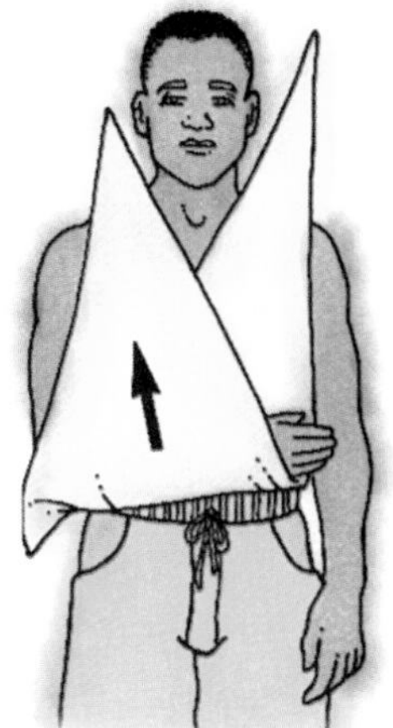

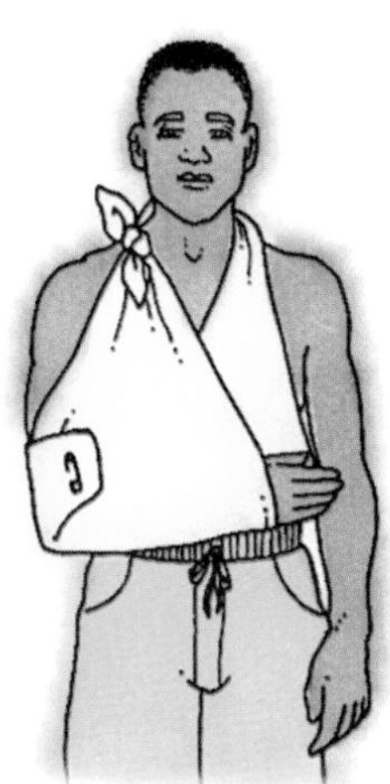

Arm sling

Finger bandages

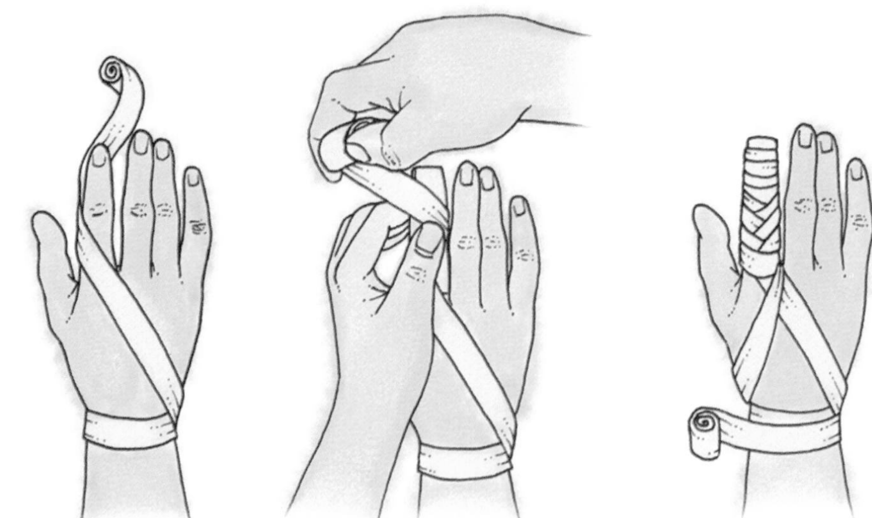

Ankle bandages

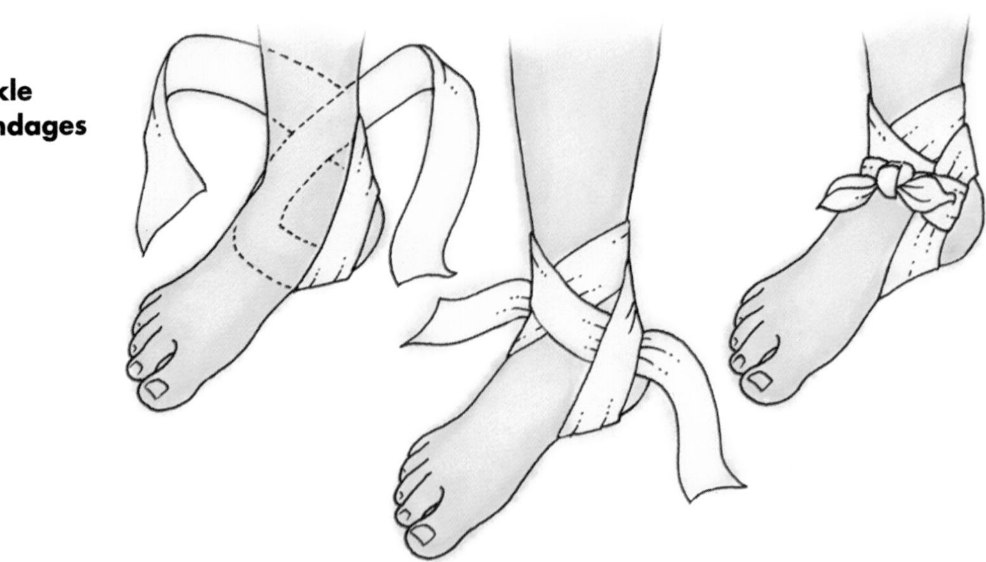

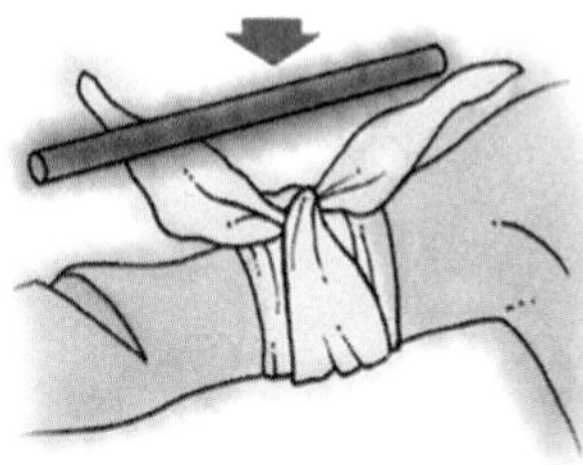

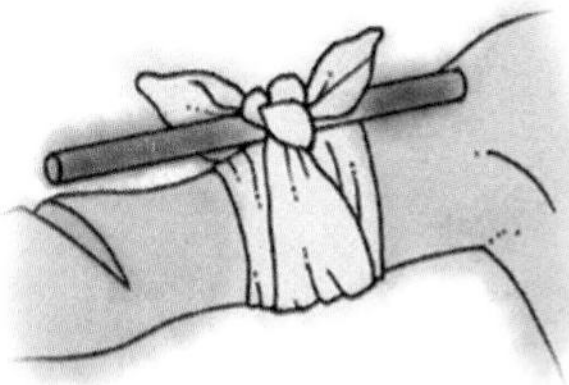

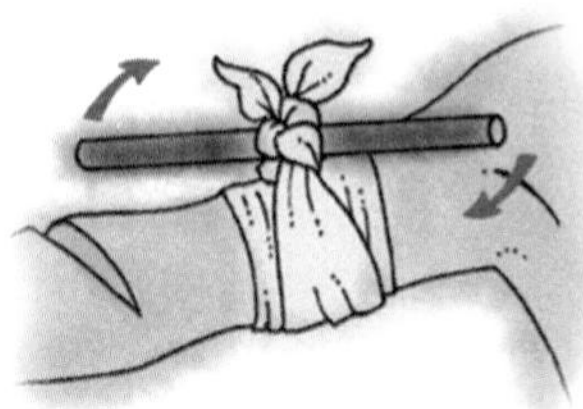

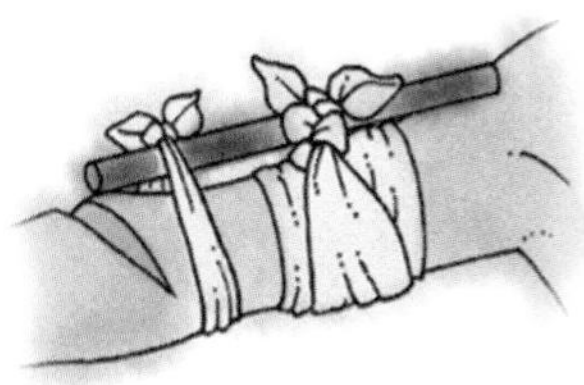

The four steps in applying a tourniquet. A tourniquet should NEVER be used unless the hemorrhage is life threatening.

exactly what should be done under a large variety of emergency situations. It is available at bookstores and at the American Red Cross office nearest your home.

Poisonings

Chapter Outline

- First aid for poisonings
- Play it safe
- Specific poisons
- Five important procedures

Millions of poisonings occur each year with over 6,000 deaths, 80 percent of which are children one to four years of age. Medicines lying around the home are common causes, aspirin and iron being among the most common. Pesticides and insecticides also take their toll. The elderly are not immune, since they may forget whether they took their medications and sometimes overdose themselves. With the rampant use of addictive drugs, death from overdose is all too common.

Fortunately, deaths from accidental poisoning have been greatly reduced in recent years as a result of widespread knowledge about first-aid procedures, prompt and efficient action by physicians in general, and the development in all major cities of poison-control centers. Little children are at high risk, since the medicine cabinets and cupboards in our homes and garages have shelves that are packed with medicines, cosmetics, detergents, bleaches, stain removers, paint thinners, lacquer solvents, insecticides, garden pesticides, and liquid and powder plant foods and fertilizers. Every home should have rules for safeguarding innocent children from needless exposure.

First aid for poisonings

The emergency call. Anytime you suspect that you or someone you are with has been poisoned, place an emergency call at once for a physician, the emergency medical squad of the fire department, or the **poison-control center** of the nearest city. In the United States and Canada, the number of your local fire department is usually listed with other emergency numbers on the inside front cover of your telephone directory.

If you are the one who will give immediate first aid till help arrives, try to find someone else to make the call. Give the name, address, telephone number, and the precise location of the victim. Provide as much information as possible as to the nature of the poison, including its name, and if you

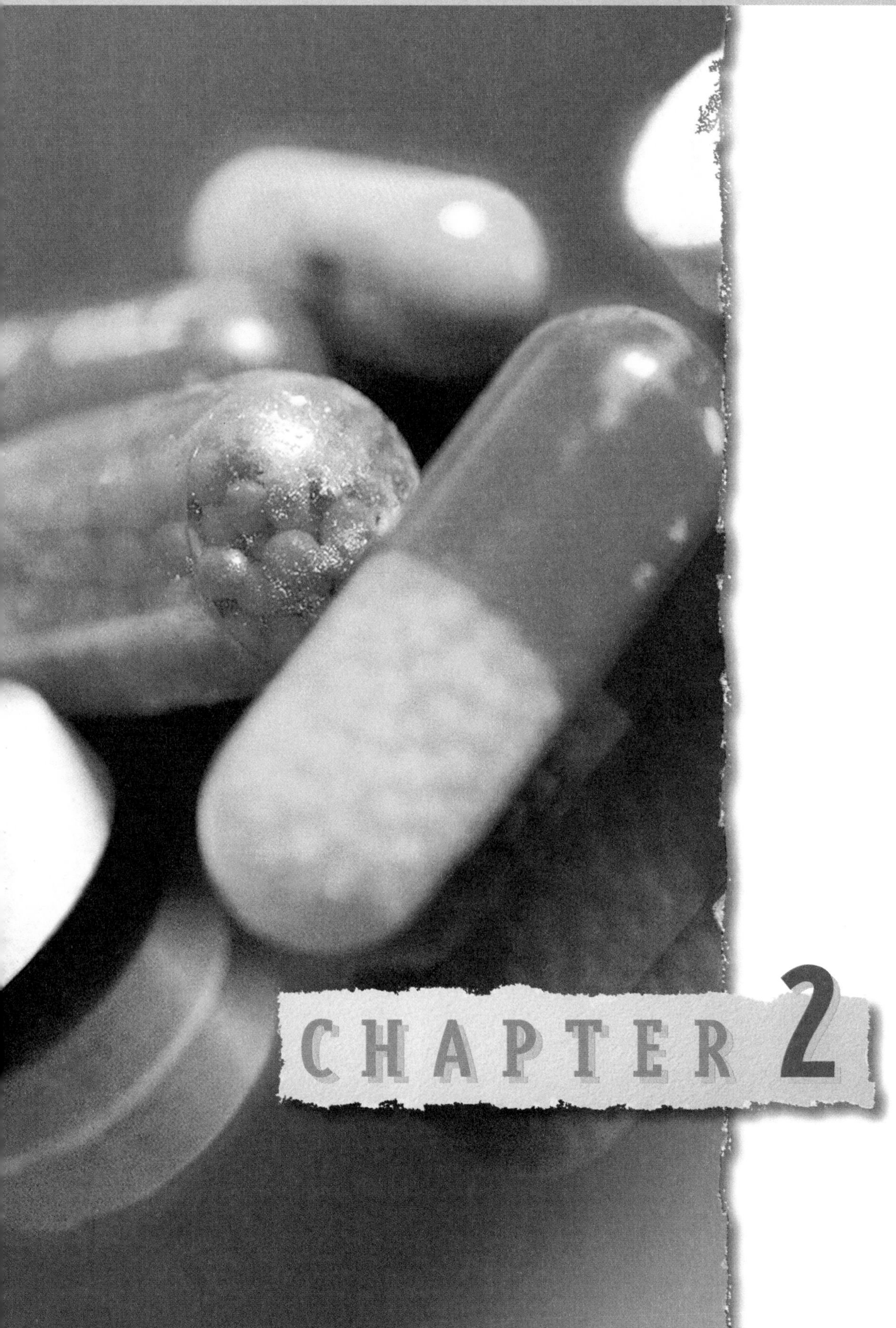

CHAPTER 2

Play it safe

The American Medical Association recommends the following:

1 Keep all drugs, poisonous substances, and household chemicals out of the reach of children. (And remember children can climb.)

2 Do not store non-edible products on shelves that are used for storing food.

3 Keep all poisonous substances and drugs in their original containers; don't transfer them to unlabeled containers.

4 When medicines are discarded, destroy them. Don't throw them where they may be reached by children or pets. Flush them down the toilet, when possible.

5 When giving flavored or brightly colored medicine to children, always refer to it as medicine—never as candy.

6 Do not give or take medicine in the dark.

7 *Read labels* before using chemical products.

have the package or bottle, the suggested antidote.

Carefully observe the victim so that you can report all signs and symptoms that might help the first-aid personnel or your physician to advise you. Especially watch for the following: The victim's skin—whether it is dry or moist, cold or clammy, ruddy or blue-colored; the type and rate of his respiration; whether he is vomiting or having diarrhea; whether he is in pain, and if so, where; and his mental state—whether he is confused, conscious or unconscious, or convulsing. Request instructions on caring for the victim until help arrives, or while you are taking him to the emergency room.

Poisons injected through the skin. This includes bites or stings from animals (dogs, cats, squirrels, bats), reptiles (snakes), and insects (spiders, bees, wasps). See pages 30-37.

Poisoning by skin contact. Many chemicals not only injure the skin but can be absorbed into the bloodstream and affect body organs. See pages 19-25.

Poisoning by inhalation. Remove a person who has breathed a poisonous gas (such as carbon monoxide) to a place where the air is fresh and administer artificial respiration if necessary. See page 26.

Poisoning by mouth. In ALL cases call for trained help. Gather all the information you possibly can about the identity of the substance, including the container, the label, and any remaining poison.

The two principles underlying any poison treatment are to **decrease further damage** and, when possible, to **remove the poison**. Dilute the poison with water or milk. If the substance is noncorrosive and the victim is conscious, you should induce vomiting (see page 67). However, if the substance that was swallowed burned on the way down, it will also burn on the way up, and you should not induce vomiting.

Specific poisons

Corrosive agents—strong acids and strong alkalis

Do not induce vomiting. Corrosive agents include strong acids (battery acid, soldering compounds, toilet cleaners), strong alkalis (lye, ammonia, dishwasher detergents, oven cleaners). These cause severe damage to the mouth, esophagus, and stomach, with excruciating pain and rapid onset of shock. **Take the victim to a hospital emergency room immediately.**

Petroleum products

Do not induce vomiting. Petroleum products that are frequently found in the home or garage include gasoline, kerosene, benzene, naphtha, turpentine, paint thinners, furniture polishes, lacquer solvent, and carbon tetrachloride. All of these substances should be used in well-ventilated areas. Breathing "dry cleaning solution" or carbon tetrachloride is highly toxic to the liver. Victims who have swallowed any of these chemicals suffer severe pain and distress. If vomited and inhaled, they may cause a serious chemical pneumonia. **Take the victim to a hospital emergency room immediately.**

Inhaling some of these volatile substances rapidly transfers them to the blood. Young people occasionally "sniff" glue, lacquer thinner, nail polish, and cigarette lighter fluid for a transitory "high." However, these substances irritate the heart, injure the lungs and liver, and if not fatal, may result in permanent damage to these vital organs.

Alcohol (ethyl alcohol; beverage alcohol)

Seek medical help. Symptoms of poisoning from acute overdose or prolonged abuse vary from deep

Many common household cleaners are highly poisonous.

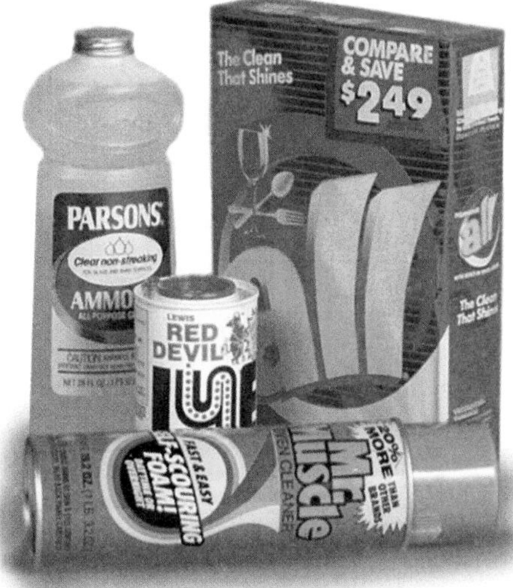

Antifreeze and paint thinners and removers contain ethylene glycol, which, without immediate medical intervention, may cause respiratory failure .

sleep, in which the pulse and respiration are good, to shock and coma. In the latter situation the skin is cold and clammy, the pulse is weak, and respiration is irregular. Death comes from failure to breathe. Keep the victim warm, see that his airway is open, and give mouth-to-mouth resuscitation if needed. If the victim is conscious, induce vomiting (see Procedure 5, page 21).

Alcohol (methyl alcohol; wood alcohol)

Seek medical help. Wood alcohol is present in paints, paint thinners, paint removers, and "canned heat." Drinking methyl alcohol causes intoxication, along with headache, pain in the abdomen, nausea, vomiting, and, because of its action on the optic nerve, permanent blindness. If the victim is conscious, institute Procedure 5. If he stops breathing, give artificial respiration.

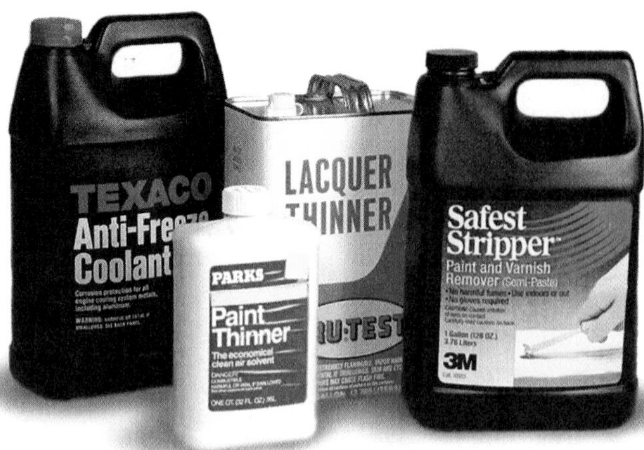

Antifreeze (ethylene glycol)

Seek medical help. Ethylene glycol is used widely in industry as a solvent, and in pure form as a coolant and antifreeze for cars. It is a sweet, colorless, slightly syrupy liquid. Taken by mouth it produces a form of drunkenness (no odor of liquor on the breath), which may develop into respiratory failure and death. If poisoning is discovered early, **institute vomiting as in Procedure 5**, page 21. Since the enzyme that breaks ethylene glycol apart also destroys alcohol, which it prefers, beverage alcohol given in large enough amounts to keep the victim drunk tends to protect the kidney from damage and may be life saving. Most of the ethylene glycol is not broken down and is excreted, being less toxic than its byproducts.

Medicinal products and drugs of abuse

Seek medical help. This is a very large class of chemical agents. While each has it own effects in the body, many can be grouped together. Some of the broad classifications, with examples, include: **sedatives** (barbiturates Seconal, Nembutal, Dolamine, and Halcion); **narcotics** (morphine, codeine, paregoric, heroin, Demerol); **stimulants** (amphetamine, cocaine, "crack," caffeine); **tranquilizers** (Librium, Haldol, Valium); and **antihis-**

Five important procedures

1.

When the victim is unconscious. Administer artificial respiration if needed (see page 6). **Do not give fluids or try to induce vomiting.** If vomiting occurs spontaneously, turn the victim's head so that the vomitus drains freely, and save it for examination.

2.

When the victim has swallowed a petroleum product. Petroleum products include kerosene, gasoline, benzine, paint thinner, fuel oil, and naphtha. **Do not induce vomiting.** Provide artificial respiration if needed. If the victim is conscious, give him a glass of milk or egg white or crushed banana to soothe the membranes.

3.

When the victim has swallowed a corrosive poison. These include strong acids or alkalis—battery acid, soldering compound, lye, caustic soda, drain and toilet bowl cleaners, and electric dishwasher detergents. **Do not induce vomiting.** The damage occurs in the mouth and esophagus. Give the victim a glass of milk, or water if no milk is available. Cream, egg white, and cracked ice are also helpful.

4.

When the poison is causing the victim to convulse. Do not prevent movements, but protect against further injury (see page 63). Loosen the clothing around the victim's neck. Keep your fingers out of victim's mouth to avoid being bitten. **Do not give fluids or try to make the victim vomit.** If vomiting occurs spontaneously, turn the victim's head so the vomitus drains freely, and save it for examination.

5.

When the victim is conscious, is NOT convulsing, and has NOT swallowed a petroleum product or a corrosive poison. Take the following steps: (1) Dilute the poison in the victim's stomach by having him drink milk or water.
(2) Induce vomiting to empty the stomach, and collect the vomitus. (3) If it is available, give activated charcoal to absorb any poison that remains.

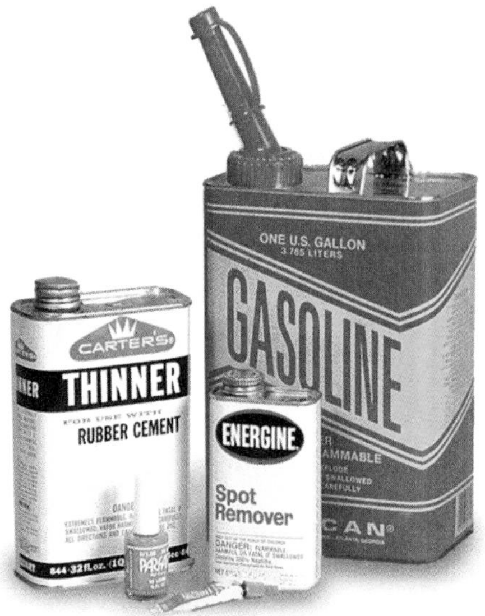

Petroleum products contain carbon tetrachloride which is highly toxic to the liver.

tamines (Clor-Trimeton, Benadryl).

The symptoms observed are: with **sedatives, narcotics, tranquilizers, antihistamines**—decreasing alertness, sleep deepening into coma, failure to breathe; with **stimulants**—increased activity, wakefulness, confusion, hallucinations, delusions, antisocial behavior.

Seek medical help first. For those who are depressed, if conscious, institute Procedure 5, page 21. If respiration fails—as in cases of severe overdose—give mouth-to-mouth resuscitation. Keep the victim warm. For those who are excited, prevent injury to themselves and others.

Aspirin and iron are the most common causes of poisoning among children. Symptoms develop slowly for both agents. **Aspirin** may cause vomiting, sweating, fever, mental confusion, unconsciousness, or convulsions. **Iron**, because of its corrosive action on the digestive tract, results in vomiting, diarrhea, abdominal pain, cyanosis (bluing of the skin), and shock. **Seek medical help immediately.** If the intake is discovered early, institute Procedure 5, page 21.

Iodine and iodine-containing preparations (Betadine) are commonly used as antiseptics for minor cuts and breaks in the skin. When swallowed, the victim may experience nausea, vomiting, painful urination, blood in the stools, and sometimes convulsions. The mouth is stained brown, and the vomitus is yellow or blue.

Seek medical help. Give plenty of fluid—milk, barley water, a starch solution, or a thin mixture of flour and water. Institute vomiting using Procedure 5, page 21.

Hair removers (depilatories)

Preparations for removing superfluous hair commonly contain thallium acetate, which is highly toxic; or barium sulfide and sodium sulfide, which are moderately toxic. Children who drink these products are the usual victims. The symptoms, which appear several hours later, include abdominal pain, vomiting, and diarrhea, which may be bloody. Damage to the nervous system causes unusual symptoms: drooping of the eyelids (one or both), crossing of the eyes, facial paralysis, and possibly delirium and convulsions. The liver and kidneys are injured.

Seek medical help. If the victim has not vomited, give several glasses of milk and induce vomiting as in Procedure 5, page 21. Give plenty of water to reduce kidney damage. Keep the victim warm,

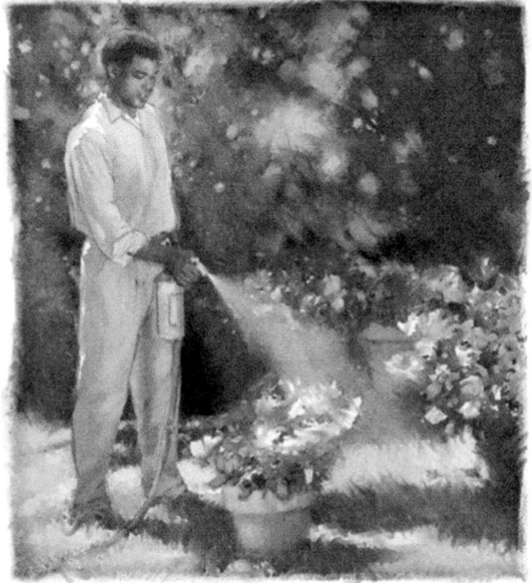

combat shock, and take him to the hospital.

Pesticides

Pesticides include a large group of generally highly toxic compounds that are commonly found in the garage, storeroom, or barn. Poisoning by pesticides can occur in one of three ways. Since they are applied as dusts and liquid sprays, they can be inhaled, either in powder or in droplet form. They may come in contact with the skin, from which many can be readily absorbed. They can also be swallowed. They kill pests by deranging certain vital processes (enzymes) within the organisms, and they can derange similar processes in the human body.

Most pesticides used today fall into one of two groups: (1) **chlorinated organic compounds** such as aldrin, benzene hexachloride, chlordane, DDE, DDT, DFDT, dieldrin, heptachlor, lindane, methoxychlor, and toxaphene; and (2) **organic phosphate compounds** such as malathion, parathion, EPN, TEPP, and OMPA.

Medical help should be sought immediately for a pesticide poisoning victim.

The symptoms of poisoning from **chlorinated compounds** include aching limbs, nervous irritability, mental confusion, muscle twitching, convulsions, and unconsciousness. Brain and liver damage may occur if treatment is delayed. The symptoms of poisoning from **phosphate compounds** include dizziness, tightness in the chest, and small pupils. About two hours later there develop nausea, vomiting, abdominal cramps, diarrhea, and muscular twitching. This may progress to convulsions, unconsciousness, and death.

Seek medical help. Use rubber gloves while removing contaminated clothes. Wash all skin areas exposed to the pesticide with soap and water. If the victim is conscious, give him several glasses of warm water and induce vomiting as in Procedure 5, page 21. If respiration fails,

While each medical product has its own effects on the body, many can be grouped together as sedatives, narcotics, stimulants, tranquilizers, or antihistamines.

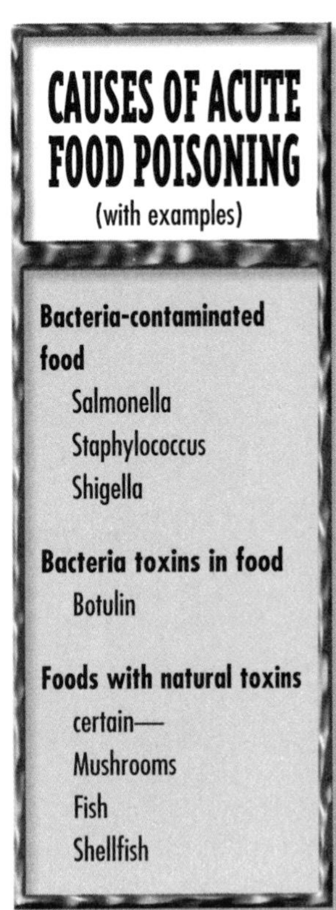

CAUSES OF ACUTE FOOD POISONING
(with examples)

Bacteria-contaminated food
- Salmonella
- Staphylococcus
- Shigella

Bacteria toxins in food
- Botulin

Foods with natural toxins
- certain—
  - Mushrooms
  - Fish
  - Shellfish

give mouth-to-mouth resuscitation. Certain antidotes are available, but must be given by a physician.

Nicotine, known as "black leaf 40," is a common garden pesticide. Absorption of nicotine is very rapid. It is an extremely poisonous substance, interfering with the transmission of nerve impulses and causing death through stoppage of the heart or respiratory failure. The victim experiences a hot, burning sensation in the upper digestive organs, and convulsions may occur.

Seek medical help. If the victim is conscious, induce vomiting as in Procedure 5, page 21. Give activated charcoal, or if that is not available, a strong tea. If breathing stops, start artificial respiration. If the heart stops, begin CPR. Atropine is lifesaving but must be given by a physician.

Insecticides and rodent poisons

Substances used to kill rodents include phosphorus, arsenic, cyanide, strychnine, and warfarin (Coumadin). Many of the aerosols used to kill flies, wasps, gnats, and ants contain petroleum distillates (see pages 19-21).

Arsenic is also an active ingredient in insecticides and certain crop sprays. Early symptoms are similar to those of food poisoning, with vomiting, diarrhea, and severe abdominal cramps. Later there are muscle cramps, kidney failure, unconsciousness, convulsions, and collapse.

Seek medical help. If poisoning is detected early, institute vomiting as in Procedure 5, page 21. Your physician will administer dimercaprol (BAL), an effective treatment.

Phosphorus, now outlawed in most rodent and roach poisons, is present in many fireworks and causes burning in the mouth, esophagus, and stomach with nausea, vomiting, and diarrhea. The breath has a garlic odor. Damage to the liver and kidneys is extreme. **Seek medical help.** Do not give oily or fatty substances. If there has been skin contact, wash thoroughly. Keep the victim warm, and give artificial respiration if necessary. In the emergency room the stomach may be washed with copper sulfate or potassium permanganate.

Cyanide. Poisoning can result from swallowing, inhaling a vapor, or absorption through the skin of cyanide-contain-

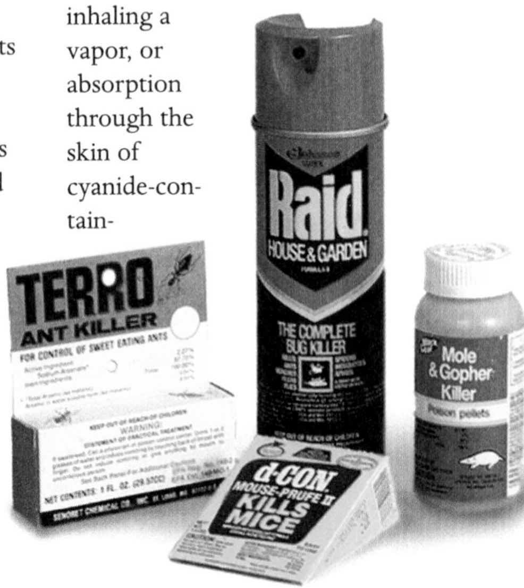

Pesticides include a large group of generally highly toxic compounds that are commonly found in the garage, storeroom, or barn.

ing preparations, including silver polish. Cyanide is extremely rapid in its action, blocking the use of oxygen, and causing respiratory failure and convulsions. Smaller doses cause difficulty in breathing, confusion, vomiting, and diarrhea. **Seek medical help.** Induce vomiting immediately by placing a finger in the victim's throat. If amyl nitrite ampoules are available (used to relieve heart cramps), break a vial and have the victim breathe the fumes. Repeat in two minutes. If the victim reaches an emergency room in time, sodium thiosulfate by vein is lifesaving.

Strychnine causes the muscles to contract, resulting in violent convulsions. Death usually is due to inability to breathe because of prolonged muscle spasms. There is no specific antidote. **Seek medical help.** Keep the victim quiet, in a darkened room. An anesthetic or a curare-like compound can be given to prevent convulsions. The stomach may be washed out and activated charcoal administered. Artificial respiration may be needed.

Coumarins (Warfarin) reduce the ability of the blood to clot, and large doses result in internal hemorrhages. Rodents bleed internally and dehydrate (desiccate). **Seek medical help.** If the poisoning is discovered early, institute vomiting as in Procedure 5, page 21. In the emergency room a vitamin K product is given orally, and intravenously if needed. In critical situations a fresh whole blood transfusion may be lifesaving.

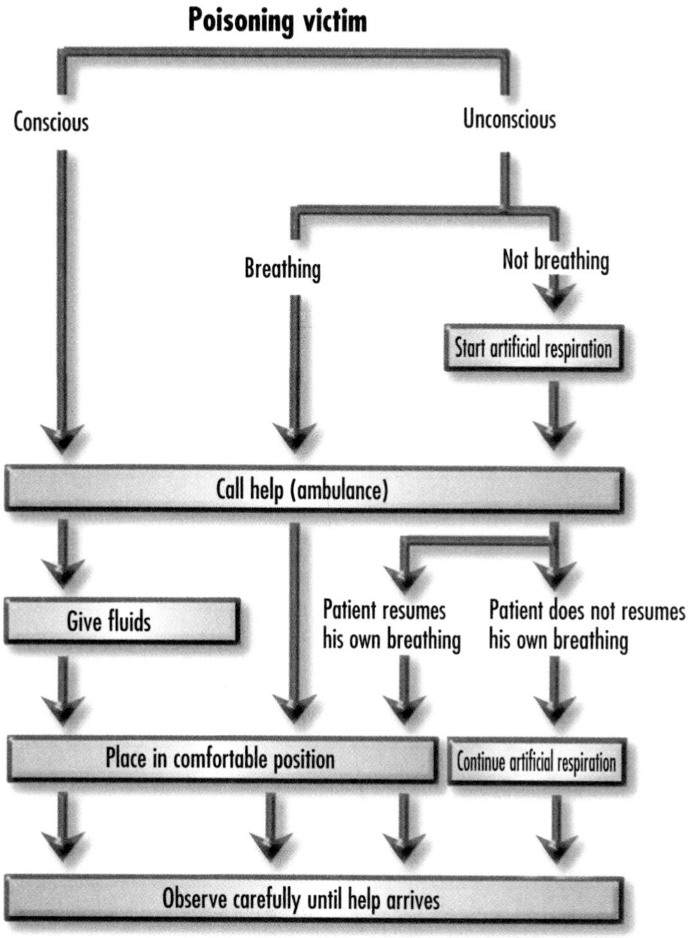

Steps in the care of a victim of poisoning.

Food poisoning

Food poisoning results from eating (1) food which has been contaminated by toxic bacteria, (2) food containing a bacterial toxin, or (3) a food naturally containing a poisonous substance.

Toxic bacteria. The illnesses and treatment of infections of this

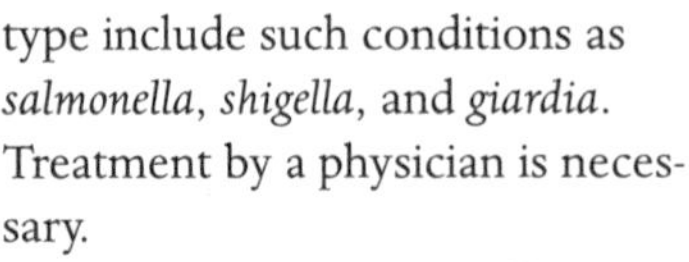

Each year some two million cases of Salmonella infection occur in the United States. It is spread by infected poultry, eggs, raw milk, and meat.

type include such conditions as *salmonella*, *shigella*, and *giardia*. Treatment by a physician is necessary.

Bacterial toxin. An illness called **botulism** is caused by a toxin produced by a germ that is often present when food is improperly canned, or when it is smoked and preserved without cooking. Examples include canned garden vegetables, turkey loaves, and salted air-dried white fish. The toxin prevents nerve conduction. Symptoms, which occur within eighteen hours after the food is eaten, include visual disturbances and difficulty in talking and swallowing due to muscle weakness. If untreated, paralysis of the breathing muscles will cause death in 70 percent of victims. **Seek medical help.** Artificial respiration may be required. The victim should be hospitalized. An antitoxin is available and can be lifesaving.

Toxic foods. Several varieties of mushrooms contain highly toxic substances. Symptoms, which develop some hours after the mushrooms have been eaten, include vomiting, abdominal pain, diarrhea, prostration progressing to shock, convulsions, unconsciousness, and death in about half the cases. **Seek medical help.** If discovered early and vomiting has not yet occurred, induce vomiting as in Procedure 5, page 21. The victim should be hospitalized, where he will be treated for shock and respiratory failure should these develop.

Carbon monoxide gas

Some 10,000 cases of carbon monoxide poisoning are reported each year in the United States. Of these, one in seven die accidentally, and one in four are suicide deaths. Carbon monoxide is found in automobile exhaust fumes (reduced appreciably by catalytic converters), inefficiently burning and poorly vented furnaces and stoves (both gas and wood), and in smoke. The gas is colorless and odorless. Hemoglobin's affinity for carbon monoxide is 200 times greater than for oxygen. It not only displaces oxygen from this pigment-carrying protein, but also retards the release of oxygen in the tissues. Death is due to oxygen depletion.

Symptoms may come on gradually with headache, faintness, dizziness, weakness, difficulty in breathing, and vomiting, followed by collapse and unconsciousness (coma). Exposure to high concentrations results in unconsciousness, seizures, and death. In a small number of victims the skin has a cherry-red

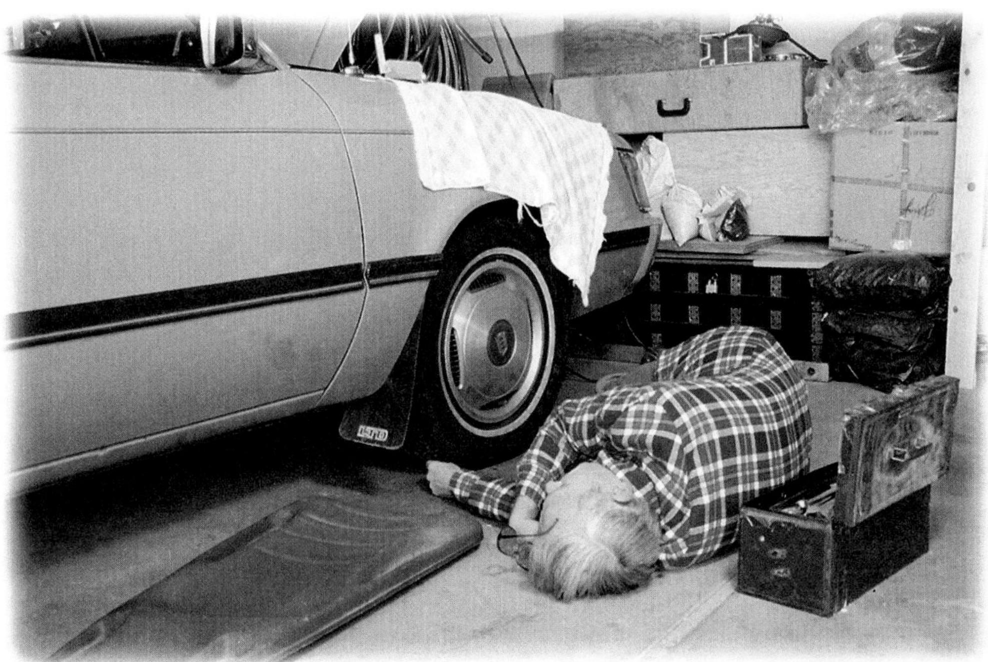

Auto exhaust fumes contain carbon monoxide, which is a deadly poison.

appearance. Prolonged exposure may cause permanent damage to the central nervous system and other organs of the body.

Seek medical help. Call the fire department or police emergency squad. The victim must be removed from the source of poison gas and given 100 percent oxygen, if available, to breathe. Should recovery occur, he should be kept at complete rest for several hours.

First aid

Chapter Outline

Several basic emergency procedures, needed from time to time in rendering first aid to someone who is badly injured or seriously ill, were presented in an earlier chapter (see page 4). In this chapter a large number of problems that require first aid will be discussed in detail. For convenience they are grouped by categories.

Every family should have at hand a book on emergency procedures and first aid, available in most bookstores. These books concisely present what should be done under a large variety of emergency situations.

It is advised that you be trained in these procedures by taking a course offered by the American Red Cross or a local hospital. The outline below, because of the limitation of space, cannot provide every detail that you might require, but it will help you recall the procedures you have learned.

In this section the various problems you might encounter, which might require first aid, are, for the sake of simplicity, placed in groups.

Allergic reactions

Asthma attack

An asthmatic attack occurs when the air passages in the sufferer's lungs (bronchi) are narrowed as a result of contraction of the bronchial muscles, the swelling of the lining membrane, and the outpouring of mucus. The attack is triggered by sensitivity to some substance, emotional stress, or vigorous exercise. The symptoms of an asthma attack include difficulty in breathing out (exhaling), tightness in the chest, and wheezing.

First aid

- Remove the asthmatic from any obvious cause of the problem that may be present, such as smoke, pollens, paints, per-

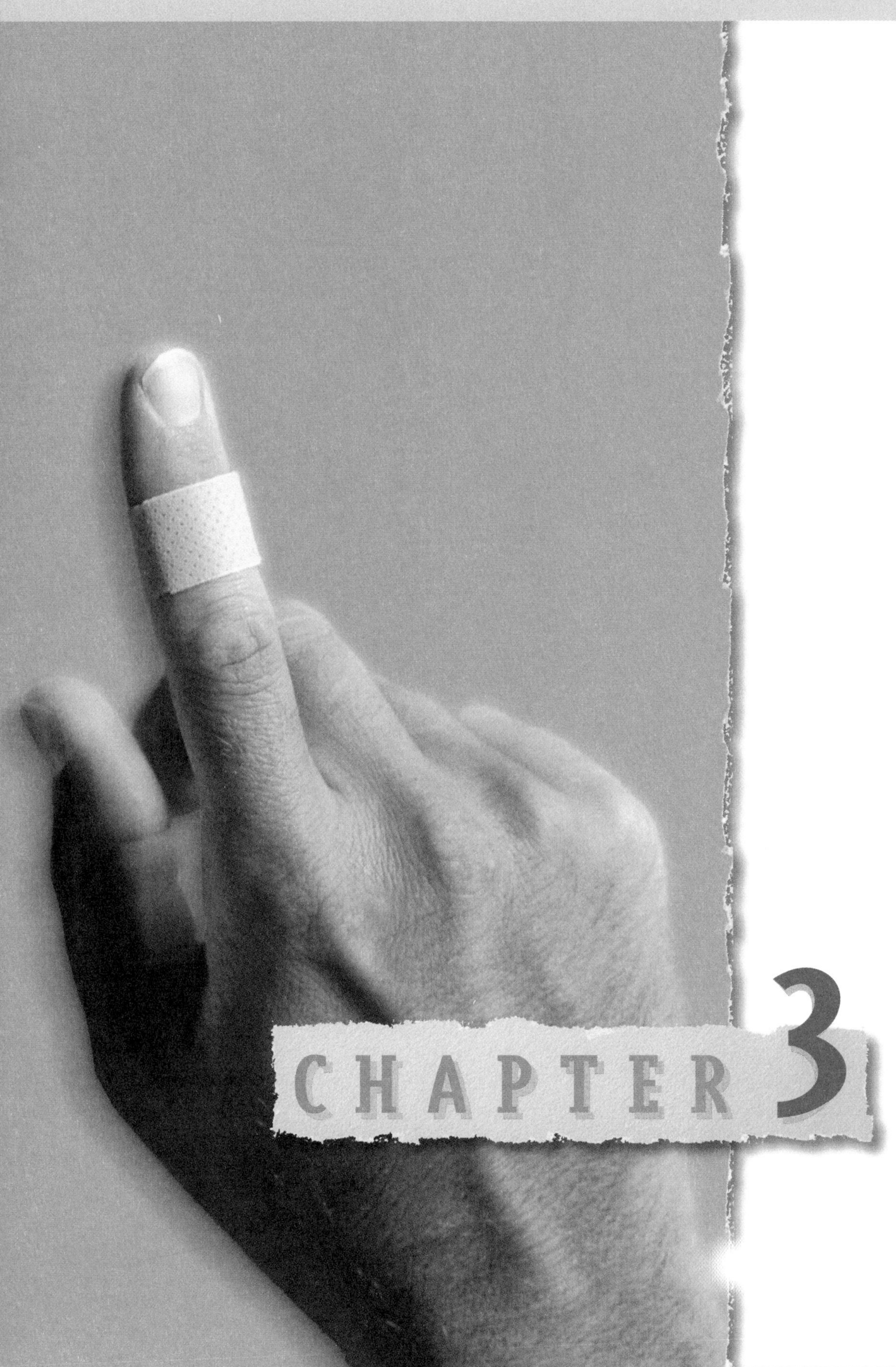

CHAPTER 3

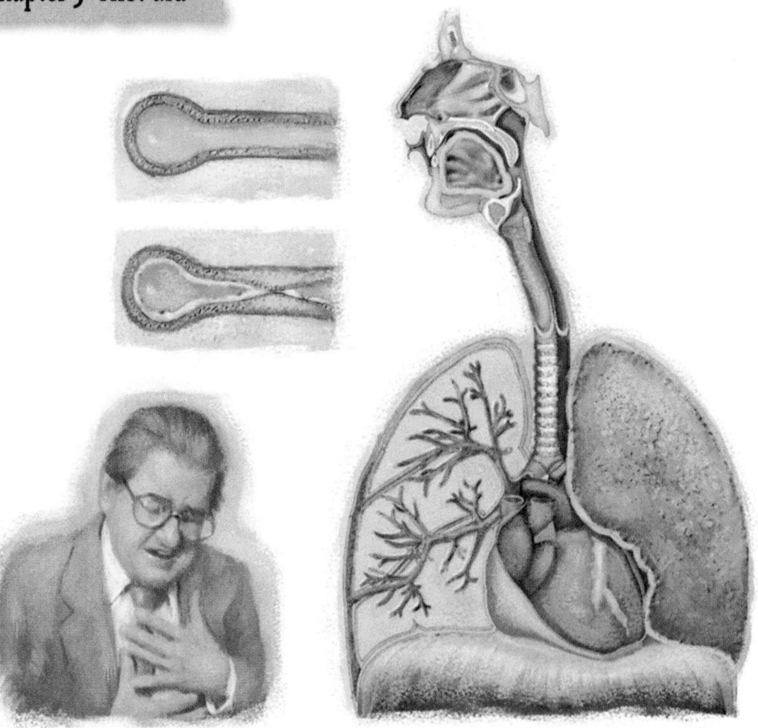

An asthmatic attack occurs when the air passages in the sufferer's lungs (bronchi) are narrowed as a result of contraction of the bronchial muscles, the swelling of the lining membrane, and the outpouring of mucus.

fumes, dust, animal dander, and molds.

- If the asthmatic has had an attack before, use the medication that was provided. Preparations are available that can be purchased over the counter. These include antihistamines and inhaled bronchodilators.
- If the attack is mild, a warm drink or steam inhalation may bring relief.
- If the attack is severe, call a physician or go to an emergency room.
- Usually, the best position for the asthmatic is sitting up and leaning slightly forward. Medications are available (adrenalin, norepinephrine, aminophylline, steroids), and a physician can decide which one is best.

Bites

Animal bites

Animal bites may result from household pets or from wild animals such as bats, foxes, squirrels, possums, skunks, and others. A bite may be superficial, such as a scratch or abrasion from the tooth or claw of a household animal, or it may be deep—a puncture wound or large laceration from a domestic or wild animal, possibly transmitting tetanus and rabies.

Plant allergies

The three most common plants to which many people are sensitive are poison ivy, poison oak, and poison sumac. The infected area of the skin becomes inflamed, swollen, and covered with blisters, and there is intense itching. A waxy or resinous material causes the irritation. Extracts of these plants have been prepared as vaccines, which for some people are helpful in preventing the problem.

First aid

- The waxy or resinous material that causes the irritation can be removed with soap and water, or it can be destroyed by washing with salt solution or Epsom's salt solution (1 T magnesium sulfate per quart or liter of water).
- Once blistering has occurred, apply dressings wet with saturated solutions of either magnesium sulfate, or baking soda (1 T per quart or liter of water).
- Cover dressings with a piece of plastic to retain moisture. Topical steroid creams will give comfort when blisters begin to dry. Over-the-counter preparations are available at a pharmacy.
- Avoid scratching, as ruptured vesicles spread the rash. Should the lesions become infected, the victim may develop a fever. If the lesions are severe and involve the eyes, mouth, or sex organs, consult a physician immediately.

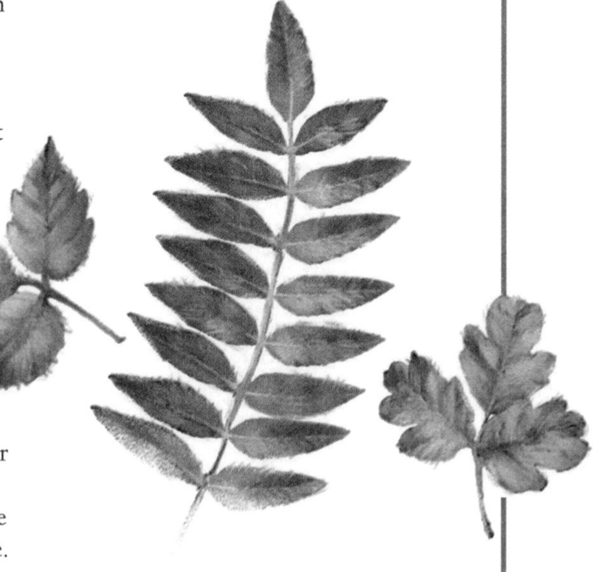

First aid

- Wash a **superficial bite** with soap and water, and apply an antiseptic (hydrogen peroxide) or antibiotic ointment. Should any lesion show signs of infection, see a physician. A tetanus shot and an antibiotic may be indicated.
- A **deep bite** should be cleaned with soap and water, and you should go to an emergency room or to a physician. He will give you a tetanus shot, and if the animal inflicting the wound cannot be found, the physician may recommend immunization against rabies. Any bite on the hand should be seen by a physician. See below.

It is extremely important to get the victim of a snake bite to a hospital as soon as possible, even if no symptoms develop.

Human bites

All human bites, especially on the hands, whether accidental or intentional, should be taken seriously. Microorganisms in the human mouth can cause very serious infections.

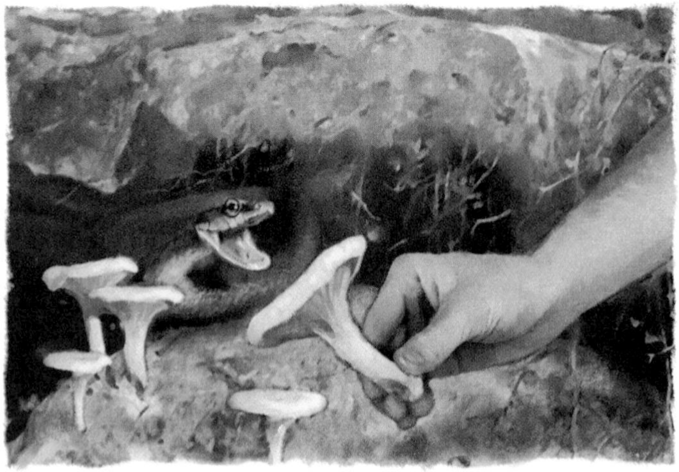

First aid

- Report to a physician immediately. Thorough cleaning and the administration of antibiotics may help prevent grave problems.

Snake bites

Poisonous snakes exist in most major countries of the world, causing many deaths, especially in children. Four kinds of poisonous snakes inhabit the United States: rattlesnakes, water moccasins or cottonmouths, copperheads, and coral snakes. The venom of different snakes varies. Venom not only damages local tissues, but also contains toxins that circulate in the blood, injuring the blood cells, the nervous system, the liver, and the kidneys.

Report all snakebites to a physician, whether from a nonpoisonous or poisonous variety. Tetanus shots and antibiotics may sometimes be given for the bite of a nonpoisonous snake. Prevention is important. Wear high boots and be on the lookout when in snake-infested territory. Do not place your hand in holes or crevices where snakes may be lying.

Antivenins for a large variety of poisonous snakes are available, but since they are specific for specific

First aid for snakebite

Poisonous or nonpoisonous

All snakebites should be medically treated. Victims should be taken to a hospital, even if the bite is only suspected.

First aid

- Act quickly. Remove the victim from the danger of a second bite.
- Get the victim to a hospital or emergency room as quickly as possible.
- Keep the victim at rest, preferably lying down. Do not allow him to move.
- Splint the limb (arm or leg).
- Keep the bite area below the level of the heart.
- Place a constricting band (*not a tourniquet*) on the heart side of the bite. *Be sure you can feel the pulse below the restricting band.* Loosen the band every fifteen minutes. If swelling occurs at the level of the band, remove and place it a few inches higher. The band should not be placed around a joint, or around the head, neck, or trunk.
- Reassure the victim.
- If shock develops, keep the victim warm.
- If breathing stops, give artificial respiration. If the heart stops, give cardiopulmonary resuscitation (CPR) if you are trained.
- If there is a snakebite kit available, follow instructions for its proper use. Antivenins are prepared from horse serum. (Hypersensitivity reactions requiring epinephrine [adrenaline] should be anticipated). The epinephrine may have to be given intravenously.

Things to remember

- It is extremely important for you to get the victim to a hospital as soon as possible, even if no symptoms develop.
- Identify the snake if possible. If it can be killed without risk, take it carefully to the hospital for precise identification.

Things not to do

- Do not give the victim food or drink, especially alcohol.
- Do not apply cold to the bitten area, such as cold compresses, ice pack, sprays, etc.
- Do not make incisions or give suction over the wound.

Symptoms

The symptoms will differ, depending on the type of venomous snake. These may include weakness, fainting, sweating, nausea, vomiting, chills, and a drop in blood pressure. There may be swelling of the injured site, drowsiness, difficulty in swallowing, difficulty in breathing, and convulsions.

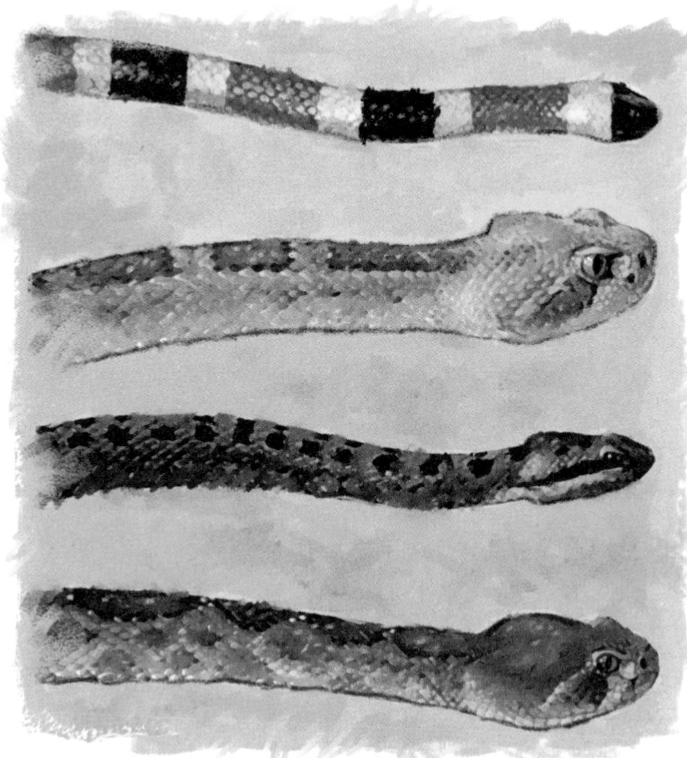

Four kinds of poisonous snakes inhabit the United States: coral snakes, rattlesnakes, water moccasins or cottonmouths, and copperheads.

snakes, identification of the snake is extremely important.

First aid

- Elevate the part of the body involved, avoid exertion, and see a physician. **Do not cut or suck or use tourniquets**.
- A summary of handling of snakebites has been prepared for your convenience. See previous page.

Spider bites

Most spiders are venomous, but lack fangs that can penetrate the human skin. The two most common poisonous spiders in the United States are the black widow (widely distributed throughout the Americas) and the brown recluse, found in the southern states. The tarantula, a large, frightening spider, does not inflict a serious bite.

The bite of a **black widow** produces sharp pain locally, followed in about thirty minutes by rigidity of the abdomen and abdominal cramps. Weakness, severe pain in the limbs, and even convulsions (especially in children) may come later.

The bite of the **brown recluse** may not become evident for hours to days. A volcano-shaped ulcer develops at the site of the bite and is accompanied with nausea, vomiting, chills, fever, and a skin rash.

The **tarantula** is not capable of instilling a significant amount of venom. The bite is painful but rarely has any serious aftermath.

First aid

- Take the victim immediately to a physician or to a hospital.
- Do not treat the site of the bite.
- In case of a black widow bite, a physician may give calcium gluconate to relax the muscle spasms, and then give the appropriate antivenin. The victim must be observed for a time for developing shock.
- For the bite of a brown recluse, some medical authorities advocate surgical removal of the

venom-infected site. Others advocate steroids. The attending physician will watch developments closely. Most lesions heal without incident.
- Tarantula bites should be observed carefully.

Tick bites

Ticks bury their heads in the skin of warm-blooded animals and drink their blood. Some ticks are harmless, while others carry a variety of diseases, some of which are serious. Do not pull a tick off, because once a tick has become imbedded, it will leave its head in the skin.

First aid

- To remove the tick, place Vaseline, oil, or a drop of gasoline, kerosene, or turpentine on the creature. This closes its breathing pores and causes it to dislodge. Or, as a last resort, grasp the tick with tweezers and rotate it counterclockwise.
- Do not touch or crush the tick with your fingers. Following removal, thoroughly cleanse the area with soap and water, then apply alcohol or hydrogen peroxide.
- Report to a physician, especially if you develop a fever within the next few days. Ticks spread rickettsial disease.

Ant bites

Bites from the many varieties of **common ants** are a frequent experience. The ant injects formic acid into the tissues. For the majority of people, the bite is limited to localized burning, itching, and swelling that spontaneously resolve in a few hours to a day.

The bite of the imported **fire ant** (present in the southern United States) evokes a much more serious response. Each bite develops into a painful pustule with localized swelling. The tissues may break down, and scarring occurs on healing.

Some people are hypersensitive to any ant bite, and for them a bite is a **medical emergency**.

First aid

- Clean bites with soap and water. An anesthetic ointment or calamine cream will provide some relief.
- Should infection develop (especially after a fire ant bite), see a physician. He may recommend an antibiotic.
- For **anaphylactic reactions** from any ant bite, *rush the victim to the nearest physician's office or hospital emergency room* for an injection of adrenalin (norepinephrine), and antihistamines given orally.

The black widow spider and tick.

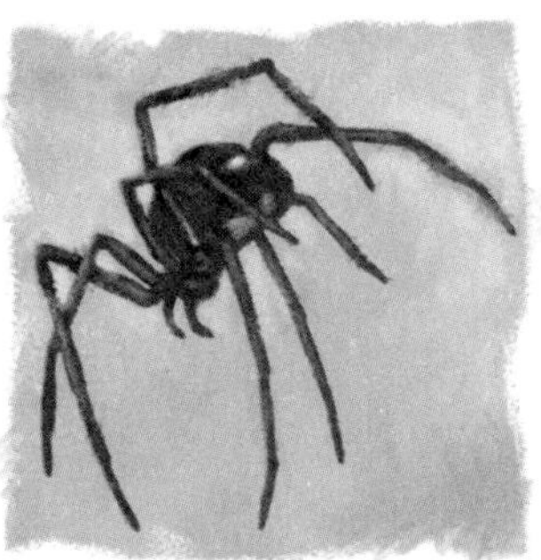

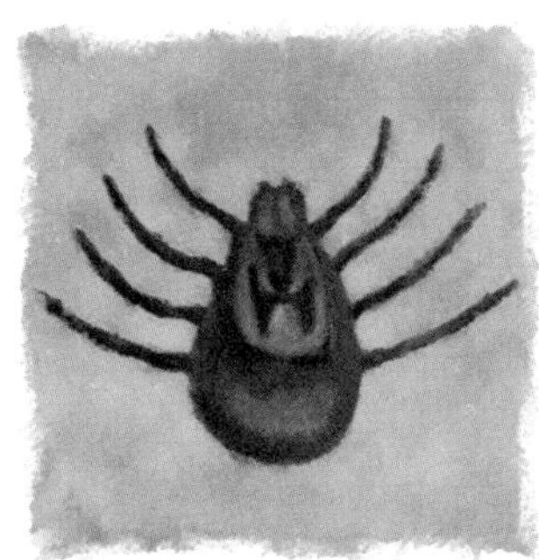

Stings

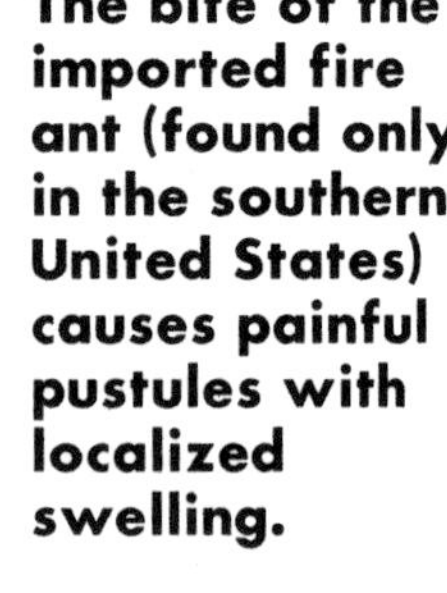

The bite of the imported fire ant (found only in the southern United States) causes painful pustules with localized swelling.

Bee, wasp, hornet, and yellow-jacket stings

The honeybee can sting only once, since it leaves its stinger in the skin. However, other stinging insects are able to sting repeatedly. Usually a single sting, although producing pain, swelling, redness, and itching at the site of the sting, is relatively harmless. On the other hand, several stings at the same time may inject sufficient venom to make the victim quite ill.

A few persons are extremely sensitive to the toxins injected by these insects and develop an **anaphylactic reaction** that may lead to shock and death in certain extreme situations.

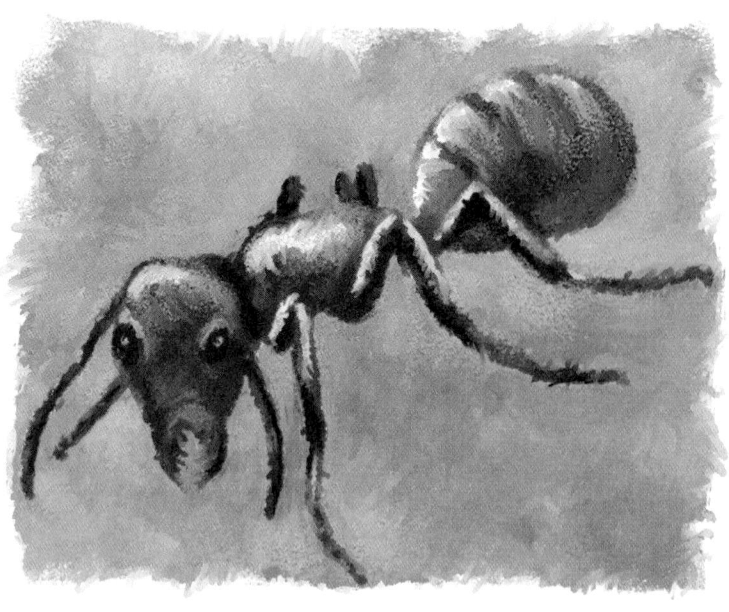

First aid

- For a **bee sting**, first remove the stinger and venom sac by lifting it off, using a knife blade or long fingernail. Do not grasp the stinger with the finger and thumb, as this will inject more venom into the wound.
- For all these stings, apply an ice pack, calamine lotion, or an anesthetic ointment to the sting site to provide relief.
- **For hypersensitive persons: If a bee-sting treatment kit is available**, give an injection of adrenalin (norepinephrine) into a muscle. An antihistamine should then be given by mouth. Watch the victim closely. If reactions develop, give an additional injection of adrenalin and take the victim to an emergency room.
- **If a bee-sting treatment kit is NOT available, rush the victim to the nearest emergency room.** If on the way to the emergency room the victim worsens, place a tourniquet about 3 inches (7.5 cm) above the sting site. Release the

tourniquet every ten to fifteen minutes. Be prepared to give artificial respiration or CPR. Treat the victim as for shock, page 10.

Scorpion sting

A scorpion resembles a small lobster and delivers its venom by a stinger at the tip of its tail. Two species of scorpions frequent the southwestern United States, the stings of which are serious but usually not fatal. The stings of scorpions in South America, Africa, and Asia are more serious and often fatal. The most serious situation is for children, and the smaller the child, the greater the danger of death.

First aid

- A physician should be contacted immediately to obtain, if possible, an antivenin, which is the only satisfactory treatment.
- Keep the victim quiet and warm. Some victims experience dizziness, vomiting, salivation, and even shock. The latter should be cared for in a hospital.

Stings by marine animals

A catfish has a barbed stinger on its dorsal fin that is strong enough to penetrate shoe leather. A jellyfish, or Portuguese man-of-war, has long, slender tentacles that stick to the skin. A stingray has a whiplike tail with the stinger located near the base of the tail. A sting from a catfish, jellyfish, or stingray causes severe pain, and may be associated with vomiting, difficulty in breathing, and fainting. The principal danger is an allergic reaction (catfish and jellyfish) or infection (stingray).

First aid

- Because of possible serious responses, it is wise to take the victim of a sting from any of the above creatures to an emergency room.
- Treat the sting of a **catfish** the same as a snakebite (see page 33).
- Remove the tentacles of a **jellyfish** by pulling them off. Some suggest rubbing them off with dry sand. The hand that is used to pull off the tentacles should be protected with a heavy towel or glove. Wash the area and then rub on alcohol. Relief may be obtained by covering the sting with a paste made from baking soda, or soaking the arm or leg in diluted ammonia water, 4 ounces to a gallon (120 ml to 4 liters), or in Epsom salts solution, 6 ounces to a gallon (180 gm to 4 liters). If the glands in the groin or armpit swell, apply an ice bag twenty minutes out of each hour.
- The barbed spine of the **stingray** should be removed by a physician. The venom is quite toxic, so the wound should be

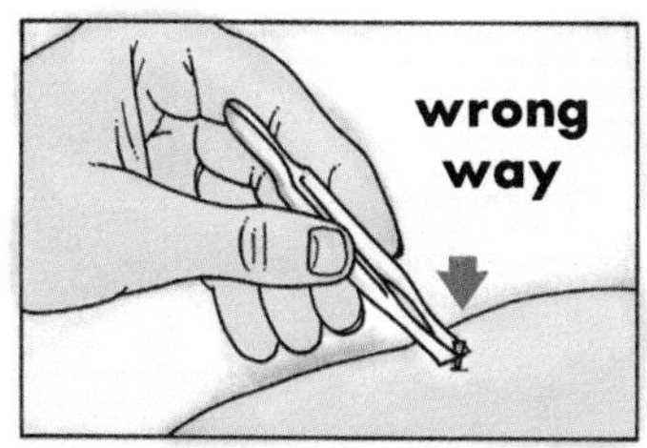

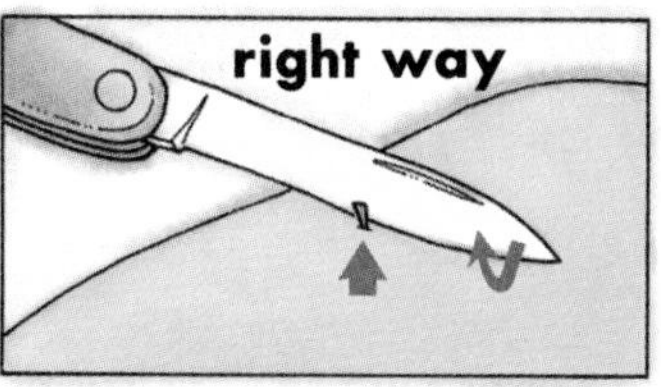

Stinger of a honey bee imbedded in the skin. Removal with forceps or finger will force venom into the skin. The stinger should be lifted off with a sharp edge (knife blade or paper edge).

Scorpion stings are serious but usually not fatal.

The venom of the stingray is quite toxic but the principal danger is infection.

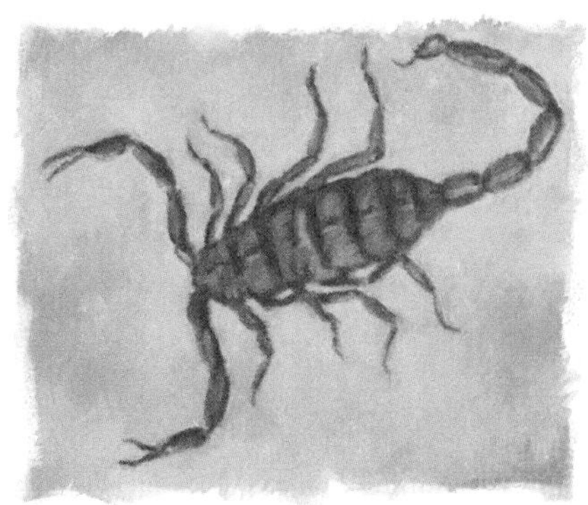

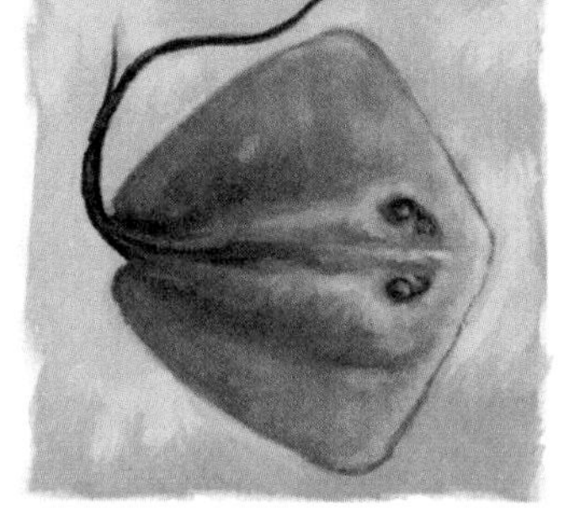

irrigated with salt water and then placed in hot water, which destroys the venom. The physician will determine whether an antibiotic is needed to prevent infection.

Burns

A burn is an injury to a tissue, usually skin or mucous membrane, caused by heat, either dry (fire, hot material) or moist (hot liquids, steam), chemicals, electricity, radiation (sun, X-ray, nuclear materials), or friction.

Some two million Americans suffer significant burns each year, of which 75,000 are serious, and of these, 10,000 end fatally. In the United States, burns are the third leading cause of accidental death.

Burns are conveniently classified as to the depth or degree of damage to the skin.

In a **first-degree burn**, only the outer layer of the skin (epidermis) is damaged. The skin is red, tender, and slightly swollen, but there are no blisters. Among the common causes of first-degree burn are mild sunburn and mild exposure to steam, hot water, or direct heat. The skin heals quickly without scarring.

In a **second-degree burn**, both the outer layer and deep layer (dermis) of the skin are injured, causing redness, swelling, blisters, severe pain, and loss of tissue fluid. Causes include severe sunburn, boiling liquids, steam, corrosive chemicals, and electricity. Extensive burns may result in systemic effects, such as shock and infections. The deep layer is not totally destroyed, so the skin will regenerate without extensive scar formation.

In a **third-degree burn**, the outer and deep layers of the skin are completely destroyed, and the burned skin is insensitive. In severe cases the underlying tissues, such as muscles, are also damaged. Causes include burning clothes, exposure to flames from fire, ignited gasoline, prolonged contact with hot objects, and electricity. The skin will not regenerate in the center, but only around the edges of the burn. Scarring may be extensive, especially when skin grafting is not successful.

The seriousness of a burn does not depend alone on whether it is a first-, second-, or third-degree burn, but also on the extent of the body's surface that is involved. As a rule, children with burns extending over 10 percent, and adults over 15 percent of their skin surface should be hospitalized. Burns on the face and inhalation burns should receive immediate medical care.

First aid

These suggestions are only for the emergency care of any serious burn. Seriously burned victims should see a physician or be taken to an emergency room.

- For a **first-degree burn**, relief of discomfort is the main goal. Immersing the burned part in cold water gives relief. Applying a non-greasy ointment containing a mild anesthetic will deaden the pain.
- For a **second-degree burn** the object of first aid is to relieve the pain, attempt to control infection, and prevent shock. Immersing the affected part in cold (not ice) water for ten to fifteen minutes most safely relieves pain. If this is not feasible, clean, laundered, and ironed cloths wrung out of ice water may be gently applied over the burn. Blot dry; don't rub. Do not use oil or greasy ointments. A small lesion may be washed with warm, soapy water. Cover the wound with a light cloth to keep it clean.
If the limbs are burned, elevate them slightly. To prevent shock, have the victim recline with his feet elevated. Keep him warm. Remove rings and bracelets that might cause problems should swelling occur. Do not break blisters.

Diagramatic views of local burns of the skin: (A) the surface layer of the skin (epidermis) has separated, and tissue fluid has accumulated to form a blister.

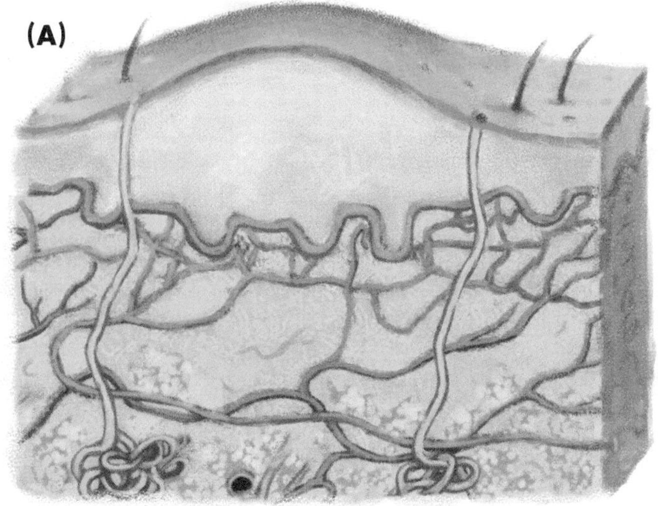

(B)

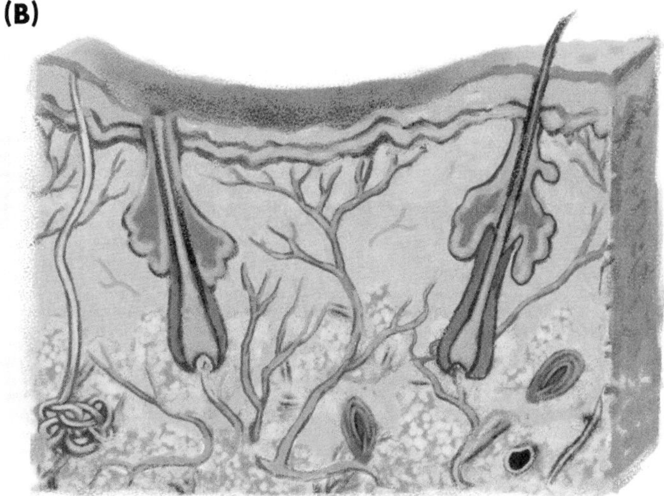

(C)

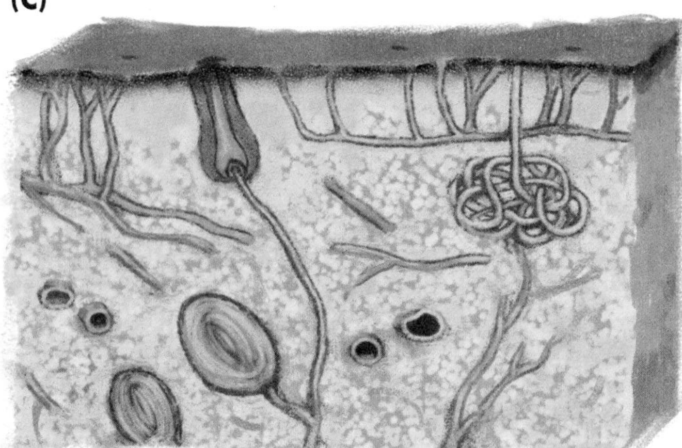

(B) A more severe burn has destroyed part of the epidermis; (C) a still more severe burn has destroyed all of the epidermis and some of the dermis; portions of sweat gland and hair follicle remain.

Give fluids frequently to replenish fluid lost from the burned area. Salt water, 1 teaspoonful to a quart (4 gm to a liter), can be given by mouth, especially if hospital care is delayed.

- For a **third-degree burn**, the general care is the same as for a second-degree burn, except that shock is much more likely. Do not attempt to clean the wound, and do not expose the burned area to cold water as this may hasten shock. Cover the burn with a sterile cloth. Watch for failure to breathe, and treat shock appropriately (see page 10).

Inhalation burns

Many severe burns resulting from explosions or blasts of hot air, together with smoke inhalation, damage the air passages and lungs, causing persistent coughing, hoarseness, and spitting of blood or particles of carbon. Swelling of the lung tissues may endanger life.

First aid

- Immediately take such victims to a hospital for continued observation, as serious problems may develop days later.

Chemical burns

In the past it was advised to immediately look for an antidote. Do not do this, as this takes time.

First aid

- Without any delay, flush the burned area with cool running water for ten to fifteen minutes. If large areas are exposed to the chemical, use a hose or shower.
- Carefully remove all contaminated clothes.
- If one eye is involved, hold the eye open, irrigate continuously with water, being careful to allow the water to run out-

ward, away from the other eye. If both eyes are affected, hold the head forward so as to permit the water to flow off the face.

- For **alkali burns of the eye**, wash as indicated above, cover with a clean, moist cloth, and go to an emergency room. A specialist should care for the victim, as serious, long-term damage may occur.
- If the chemical container carries specific first-aid instructions, follow them.
- Cover with a clean, moist cloth and take the victim to an emergency room.
- For **acid burns**, thoroughly wash the area with water, and, if available, wash with a weak solution of soda (sodium bicarbonate), 1 teaspoonful of soda to a quart of water (4 gm to a liter).
- For **alkali burns other than in the eye**, wash as above, and take the victim to an emergency room.

Radiation burns

These occur from overexposure to ultraviolet light (sun, sunlamp, welding torch), X-rays, and nuclear materials.

First aid

- For first-and second-degree burns from **ultraviolet light**, treat as for ordinary burns. For the treatment of burns in the eyes from observing arc welding without adequate protection, see your physician.
- For **X-ray** and nuclear burns, treat superficial skin burns as ordinary burns. Delayed symptoms require expert hospital management.

Acute circulatory problems

Heart attack

A heart attack may come as a surprise, or the person may have been aware of a heart problem. Heart disease is a growing health problem. While occasionally the attack is "silent," the two main symptoms of an acute heart attack are (1) pain in the chest radiating to the neck, one or both shoulders, and the upper abdomen (which is sometimes mistaken for indigestion), and (2) severe shortness of breath. There is pallor, a cold sweat, nausea (sometimes vomiting), extreme apprehension, prostration, and frequently shock.

Electrical current burns

Electrical current burns

Serious damage occurs at the point where an electric current enters and leaves the body. The damage is often greater than what appears on the surface and may not become apparent for several days. The most serious problems result from passage of the current through the chest, interfering with the heart action, and through the base of the brain, affecting control of breathing.

First aid

- If the victim is still in contact with the electric current, break the contact, using an insulated tool such as a piece of wood, or some other nonconducting instrument. Take care not to receive the current and become a victim yourself.
- Give immediate attention to the action of the heart and lungs, and if necessary, institute artificial respiration or CPR (pages 6-9).
- Call for medical help or take the victim to an emergency room.
- Minor burns can be treated as ordinary burns.

A victim of electrical shock should first be separated from the electrical current using some nonconducting instrument (wood, plastic). Otherwise, the rescuer may also become a victim.

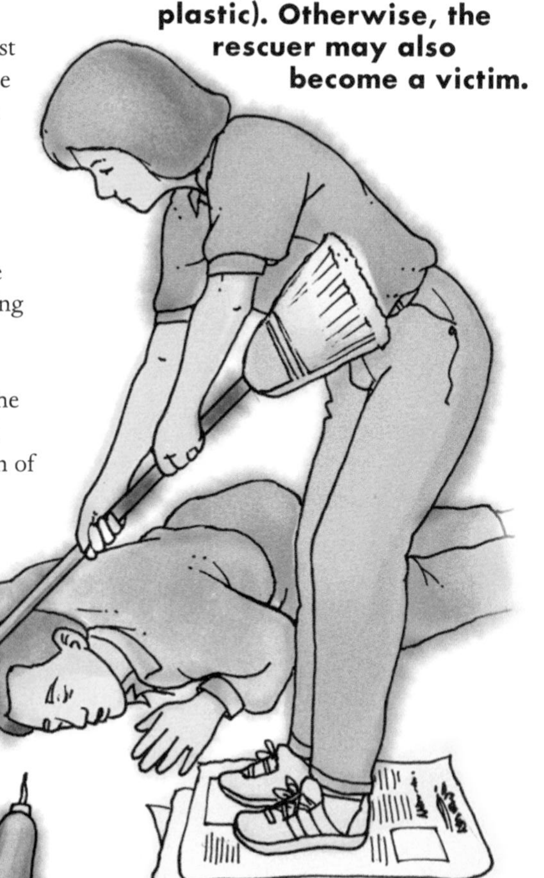

First aid

- Send someone for emergency help—paramedics or an ambulance—and notify a physician.
- Place the victim in a half-reclining position, and keep him at absolute rest. Loosen clothing around the neck.
- Should respiration stop, start artificial respiration. Should **cardiac arrest** occur (when the heart stops beating), commence CPR.
- If the victim has had previous attacks and has nitroglycerine, place a tablet under his tongue.
- When trained help arrives, follow their instructions. Allow the victim to be taken to a hospital coronary care unit.

Stroke

A stroke results from a hemorrhage into the brain tissues or a clot forming in a brain artery. Strokes may be major, usually causing serious disability, or minor, sometimes called "**ministrokes**," in which the disability is only slight, and often temporary. The indications of a ministroke include headache, confusion, dizziness, speech difficulties, memory loss, and weakness in an arm or leg. If ministrokes occur frequently, personality changes may develop.

The symptoms of a **major stroke** include weakness or paralysis of one side, difficulty in speaking

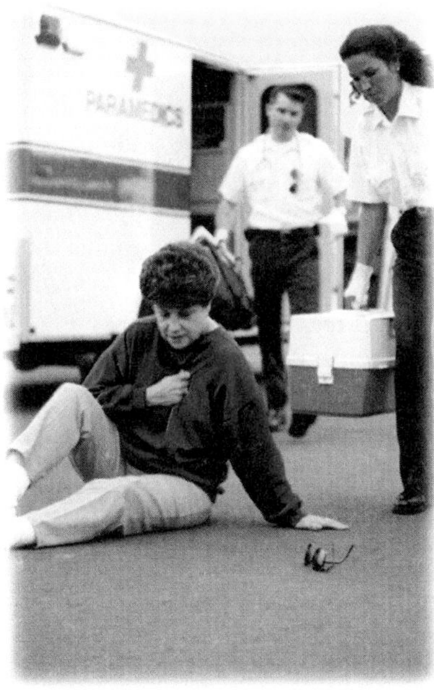

and swallowing, difficulty in breathing, and confusion or unconsciousness.

The disability can be serious and is often permanent.

First aid

- For any **stroke**, call a physician or take the victim to a hospital.
- In the meantime, keep the victim warm, quiet, and comfortable, and in a position that will allow saliva or vomitus to flow out of the mouth. If breathing stops, give artificial respiration.
- For a **ministroke**, consult a physician. In the interim, keep the victim quiet, and guard against physical exertion and injuries from falling.

Strokes may be major, usually causing serious disability, or minor, sometimes called "ministrokes," in which the disability is only slight, and often temporary.

Severe bleeding (hemorrhage)

Rapid loss of blood can lead to death in a short period. Blood lost from the circulation can be external, flowing away from the body, or internal, when blood flows into body cavities.

External bleeding may result from cuts, stab wounds, lacerations, and avulsions (when body parts are torn away). *Blood from an artery* is bright red and may come in spurts (in timing with the heartbeats). *Blood from a vein* is dark red and flows more slowly. *Blood from capillaries* is intermediate in color and oozes out.

First aid

- First, see that the victim is breathing. If necessary, give artificial respiration. If the heart stops, the bleeding will, of course, cease, but attempt CPR (page 8).
- Place a dressing or a thick cloth pad over the wound, hold it firmly in place, and apply sufficient direct pressure with the palm of the hand to control bleeding.
- If this is unsuccessful, try to put pressure on the artery above the site of the hemorrhage. Select the nearest **pressure point**, that is, where the

Two methods of controlling bleeding: (a) direct pressure over the bleeding site; (b) indirect pressure applied to the artery above the site of the hemorrhage.

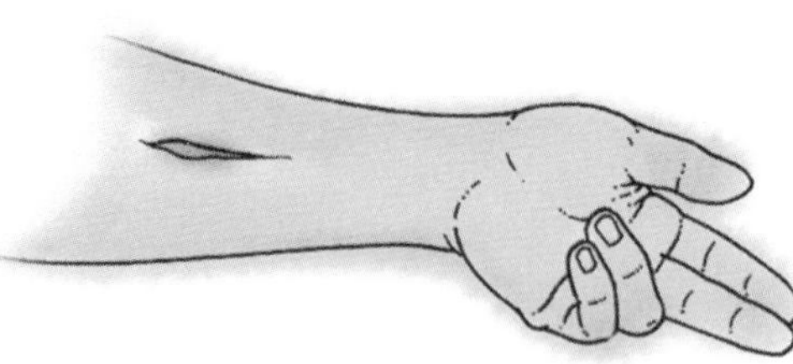

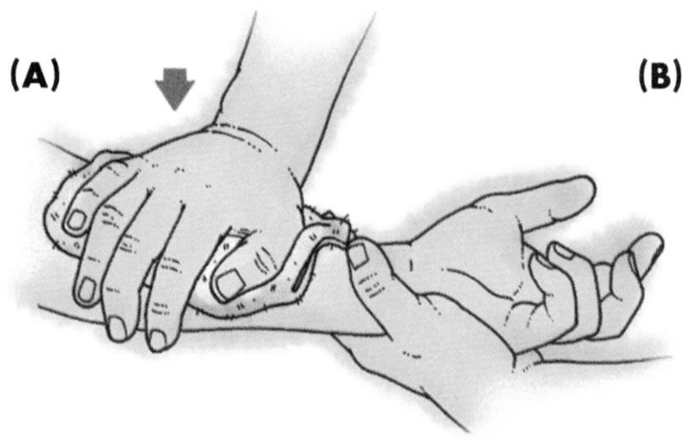

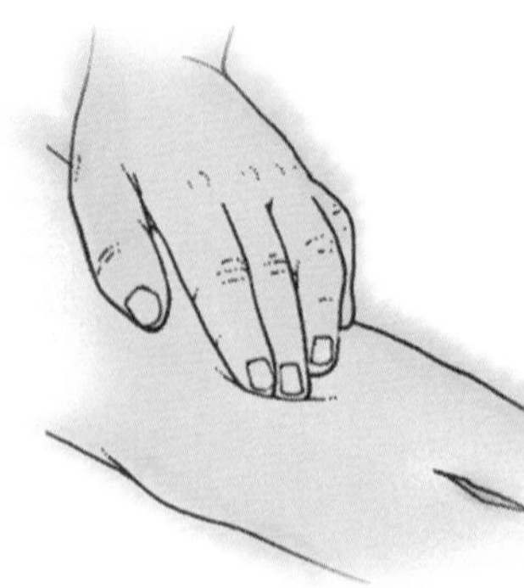

artery can be squeezed against a bone (see diagram). This technique is useful for injuries of the limbs and should not be applied to bleeding in the head or neck.

- A tourniquet should only be used when the victim would die if it were not used (see page 15 for directions). The reason for caution in using a tourniquet is that all tissues below the tourniquet will be deprived of blood, possibly necessitating the amputation of the limb.
- Treat shock should it develop (see page 10).
- Where possible, elevate the bleeding area above the level of the heart to make control of bleeding easier.
- If the victim is conscious, encourage him to drink fluids, but do not give caffeine-containing drinks, as these will raise his blood pressure, and thus increase the bleeding.
- Take the victim to an emergency room as soon as possible.

Internal bleeding may occur from a torn liver or spleen, ruptured oviduct (tubal pregnancy), stab or gunshot wound, disease within the lung, rupture of varicose veins in the esophagus, or erosion of a peptic ulcer. Bleeding from the lungs may be recognized when bright red, frothy blood is coughed up. Bleeding from sites in the stomach and intestine can be detected when blood is vomited or dark, tarry stools are passed. Signs of shock following a violent injury (such as a car accident or gunshot wound) may also indicate internal hemorrhage.

First aid

- Have the victim lie on his back and keep him warm.
- If breathing stops, give the victim artificial respiration (see pages 6, 7).
- If the victim is conscious, encourage him to drink fluids, but do not give him caffeine-containing beverages, as these will raise his blood pressure, and thus increase the bleeding.
- Take the victim to an emergency room immediately for surgical intervention.

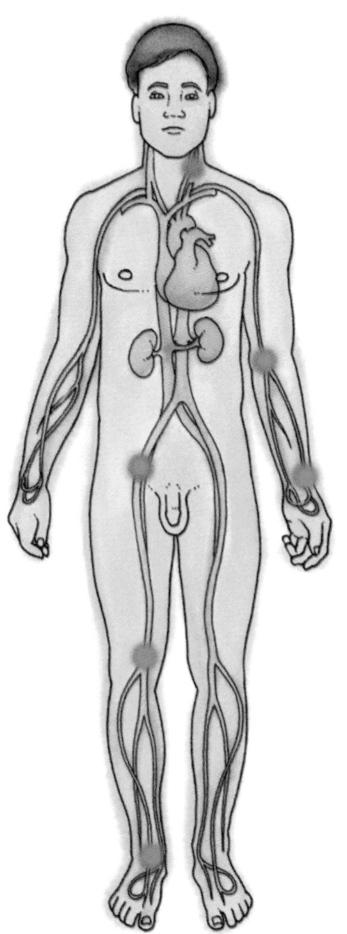

Note the various pressure points— points at which an artery is in close proximity to a bone.

Foreign bodies

Foreign objects may enter the eyes, ears, nose, throat, stomach, and skin. If simple, nonharmful procedures fail to remove the object, immediately see a physician or go to an emergency room.

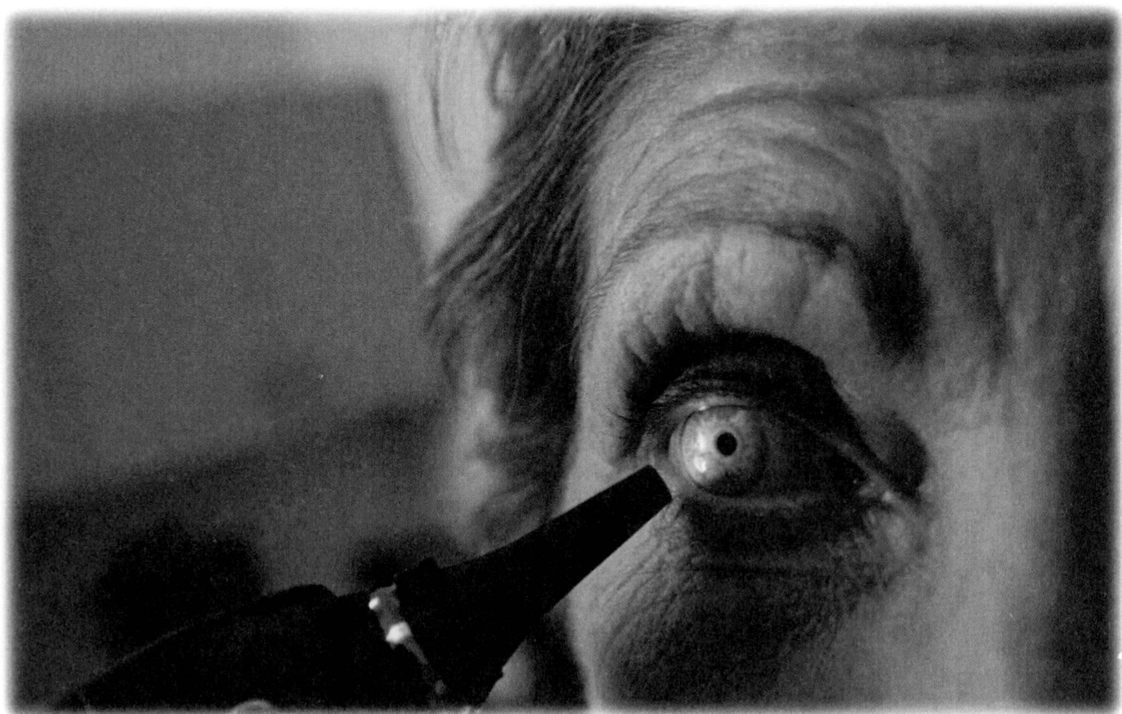

Consult a physician immediately if a splinter of steel or any other foreign material has penetrated the eyeball.

Ear canal
First aid

- If an **insect** lodges in the ear, take the victim to a dark room and shine a flashlight into the ear canal.
- If this proves to be ineffective, tilt the head so that the affected ear is up, and place a few drops of glycerine or oil (cooking or mineral) into the ear canal. This will suffocate the insect Then, tilt the head the other way and gently irrigate the ear with warm water, using a rubber syringe to introduce the water. A hard object can be sometimes dislodged by tilting the head so the affected ear is directed downward and then pulling the external ear in various directions.
- If this fails to dislodge an object that is visible from the outside, place a drop of fast-drying glue on the end of a matchstick. Gently touch the object with the glued end of the match and wait till the glue dries, then withdraw the match. The object should come with it. This should **not** be attempted if the object cannot be easily seen.
- If you are unsuccessful in removing the insect or object, see a physician.

The eye

Consult a physician immediately if a splinter of steel or any other foreign material has penetrated the eyeball. Dust particles, sawdust, and similar objects may be removed from the surface of the eye as follows.

First aid

- Do not rub. Close the affected eye for a few minutes. The extra flow of tears may wash out the particle.
- If this is unsuccessful, pull the lower lid down so its lining is visible. Have the person roll the eye up. Remove the object with the tip of a clean handkerchief or a moistened cotton swab.
- If the object is not found, grasp the lashes of the upper eyelid and draw the lid out and down over the lashes of the lower lid. Release the upper lid so that the lower lashes can brush out the foreign particles.
- If this procedure is ineffective, fill a medicine dropper with plain water or commercial eyewash solution, and, by grasping the eyelashes, draw the lids outward. Gently flush the undersurface of the lids.
- If the object still remains, invert the upper eyelid. This is accomplished by taking a wooden matchstick and pressing backward and downward on the upper eyelid while pulling the eyelid (by means of the lashes) outward and upward. Use the tip of a handkerchief to wipe the object off.
- If this is unsuccessful, or vision is blurred, or pain persists, apply an interim pressure patch to the eye and immediately take the victim to an emergency room.

The nose

Children will sometimes force beans, kernels of corn, or objects of similar size into their nostrils.

Eversion of the upper eyelid. A match or applicator stick is placed over the fold of the eyelid. By grasping the eyelashes the lid can be pulled outward and then upward.

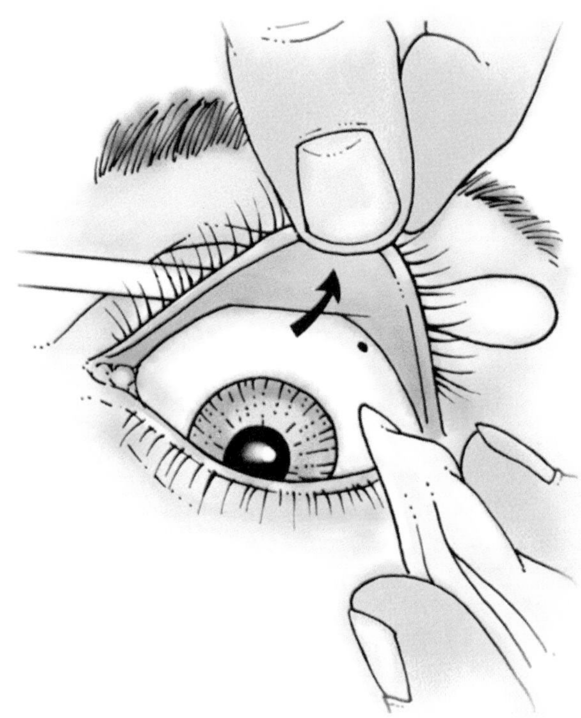

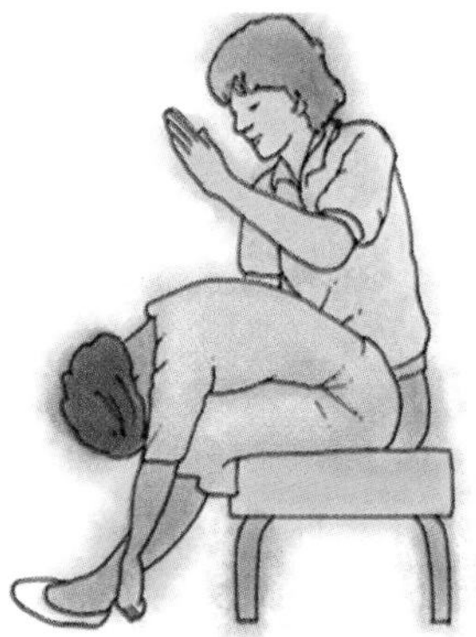

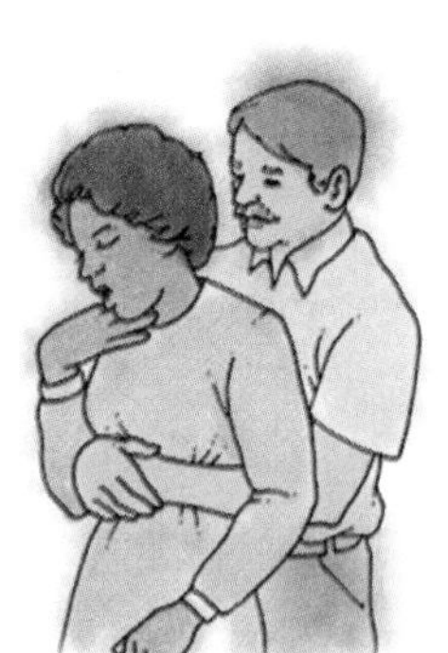

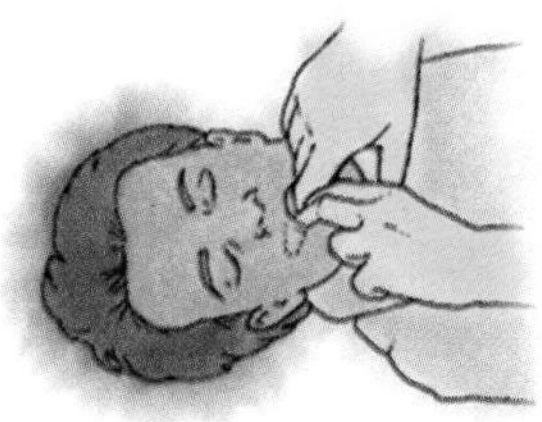

Three ways to remove an object from a blocked airway: back blows; Heimlich maneuver; and finger sweep.

First aid

- Often, simply blowing the nose, one nostril at a time, will dislodge the object.
- The nasal cavity is narrow from side to side but tall in the vertical direction. If the object can be seen by having the child tip the head backward, slip a curved loop of thin wire (a loop, **not** a bent wire with a sharp end), either over or under the object, and draw it out.
- If this is unsuccessful, see a physician.

The throat

Choking or strangling is the sixth most common cause of accidental death in the United States, causing more deaths than firearms or airplane accidents. Children often inhale an object while at play, or a bite of food too large to swallow lodges in the throat (pharynx) and completely blocks the air passageway.

First aid

- If the person has inhaled an object but can breathe, take him to an emergency room immediately. Do not attempt to dislodge the object.
- If the obstruction has completely blocked breathing and the victim is **choking** or **strangling**, attempt one or all of the following three approved procedures.

Back blows. The victim can be standing, sitting or lying on his side. Place yourself in position to deliver a series of four quickly repeated, sharp blows between the shoulder blades with the heel of your hand. The blows should be forceful enough to jar the victim's body. For an infant, support the child, face down, on your forearm or knee and deliver appropriate blows (but not as strong as with an older child or adult).

Epigastric thrust (Heimlich maneuver). If the victim is conscious, have him stand or sit. Position yourself behind him and place the thumb side of your fist against his abdomen, just above the umbilicus but below the lower end of the breastbone. Grasp your fist with your other hand, and, pulling inward, give four quick, upward thrusts. If the victim is lying on his back, straddle the hips or a thigh. With one hand on top of the other, place the heel of the lower hand just above the navel and below the breastbone. Using the weight of your shoulders, give four quick, upward thrusts toward the diaphragm.

Finger sweep. Raise the chin upwards, grasp the tongue with a handkerchief, and pull it forward. Pass the forefinger of the other hand over the tongue and along the side of the throat (not the middle, as this may push the object further in) to reach the edge of the object. With a sweeping movement, bring the object forward into the mouth.

Even after breathing has been reestablished, the victim should be seen by a physician to determine whether any tissue damage has occurred.

The stomach

It is common for small children to swallow coins, marbles, keys, seeds, bobby pins, and even safety pins. An object without sharp points will usually pass out in the stool within a day or two. The danger is that open safety pins and bobby pins may become lodged in the intestine and perforate its wall.

First aid

- See a physician immediately if an open safety pin or other sharp-pointed object has been swallowed. X-rays will reveal the object and its location. It can then be determined whether it should be removed surgically or by means of an instrument.

The skin

Usually the foreign object is a thorn, a splinter of wood, glass, or metal, or a fishhook. If the object goes underneath the fingernail or toenail or is deep in the tissues, see a physician. A booster shot for tetanus may be wise.

First aid for a splinter

- Clean the skin area with soap and water, sterilize the ends of a sharp pointed pair of tweezers and a needle, passing them rapidly through a flame, and enlarge the opening in the skin with the needle until enough of the splinter is exposed that you can grasp it with the tweezers. Withdraw it and cover the wound with an adhesive bandage.

First aid for a fishhook

- If the barb has not penetrated the skin, simply withdraw the hook.
- If the barb has penetrated the tissues, see a physician.
- If a physician is not readily available, thoroughly cleanse the site. Push the hook on through the tissue until the point of the barb appears, then cut off either end of the hook with a wire cutter and withdraw the remainder of the hook. Cleanse the wound thoroughly, apply an adhesive bandage, and see a physician for a tetanus shot. Watch for possible infection.

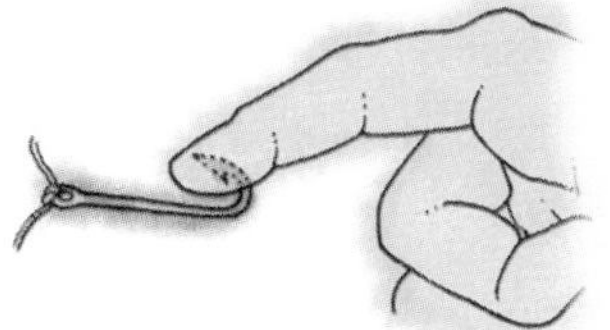

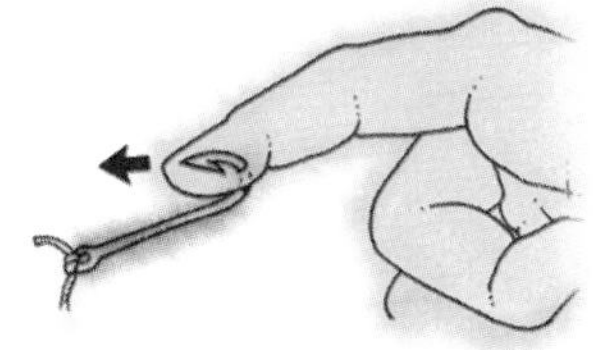

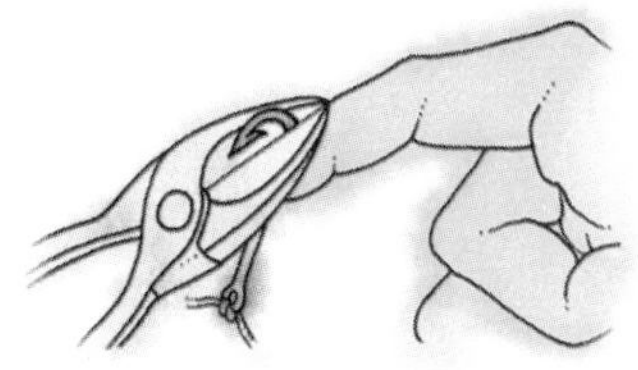

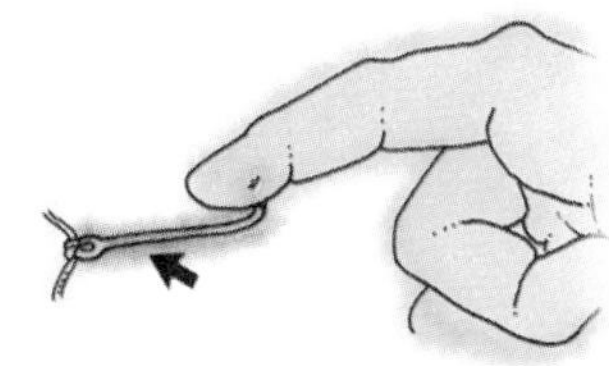

The four steps for removing an embedded fishhook.

Fractures

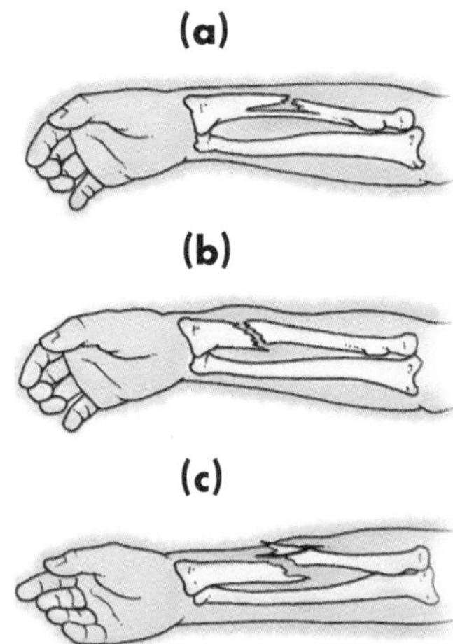

Types of fractures: (a) incomplete or greenstick; (b) closed; and (c) open

A fracture is a break in a bone. In a **simple** or **closed** fracture, the broken bone does not protrude through the skin, as it does in an **open** or **compound fracture**. A **dislocation** occurs when joint structures (joint and socket) are torn apart, displacing at least one of the bones of the joint. Broken bones and dislocated joints are painful, often misshapen, and cannot be used. A broken bone may injure adjacent structures and cause bleeding, as may happen with rib fractures.

The purpose of first aid is to protect the fracture and body structures from further injury, and, when necessary, to prepare the victim for transport to appropriate medical care and to provide whatever support care is needed.

Simple fractures

First aid

- If medical help is on the way, make the victim as comfortable as possible.
- If medical help is not immediately available or if the patient has to be moved, immobilize the fracture. Depending on the fracture site, this may be done with a sling but is usually done with a splint. Splints can be made from whatever material is available, including boards, sticks, magazines, or cardboard. The splint should reach beyond the joints above and below the injury to prevent movement of the fractured bones. An arm may be splinted to the body or a leg to the other leg (if only one is broken). Strips of cloth, neckties, leather belts, or bandages may be used to fasten the splint in place.
- It is sometimes necessary to straighten an arm or leg in order to apply a splint. Support the fracture, holding the bone above and below the break. For fractures of the lower limb, pull steadily and gently until the splint is in place.

Open (compound) fractures

First aid

- The clothing at the fracture site should be cut away and removed.
- Staunch any bleeding with a sterile (clean) pad and appropriate pressure.
- Cover the area with a clean bandage or cloth.
- If the victim must be moved, splint the fracture as necessary (see the next page).

Dislocations

These are handled as are simple fractures.

General principles of first aid care

- See that the victim is breathing, and give artificial respiration if needed. Check the pulse, and, should the heart stop, start CPR (see page 8).
- Keep the victim warm and watch for signs of shock.
- If there is severe bleeding, place a gauze or cloth pad over the wound and apply necessary pressure.
- If the conditions warrant it, call for medical assistance or an ambulance.
- Do not let the victim use or move a possible fracture, as this may make the condition worse.
- Do not try to set or reduce a fracture or dislocation.
- Do not attempt to move a victim or splint a fracture if trained medical help is on the way, unless the circumstances demand that this be done.

Special situations

Fractures of the neck, spine, head, ribs, and pelvis may require additional precautions. Fractures in these sites should be suspected after observing bumps and abrasions, abnormal positions of body parts, the type of accident, and the victim's complaints of pain, numbness, or paralysis.

Neck or spine fracture

These usually result from automobile accidents, whiplashes, falling from a ladder, jumping from too high a height, and diving incorrectly into a shallow pool.

First aid

- Keep the victim absolutely motionless. Place clothes, blankets, or any suitable materials on either side of the head or back to prevent movement.
- Move the victim only if necessary, when there is danger of fire or explosion. Obtain the help of several people to lift the victim (or to turn him when this is necessary for breathing), so that many hands, working together, prevent the back, neck, or head from bending or moving in any direction. Lift the victim onto a stretcher, board, door, or any available rigid material. If the victim sus-

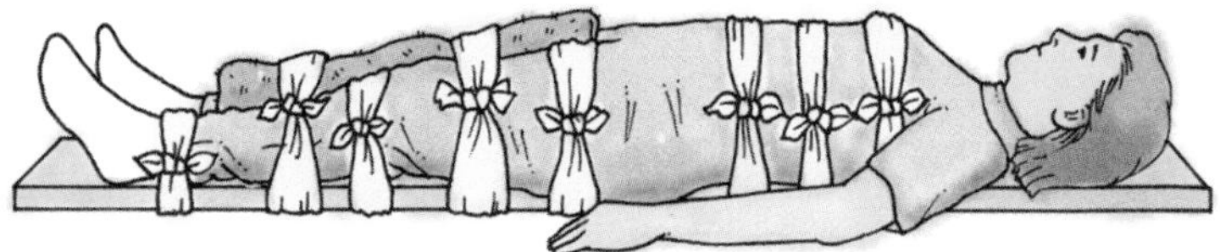

Fractures of the neck and spine require splinting to prevent any movement. A full-length board is appropriate for these and certain fractures of the lower limbs.

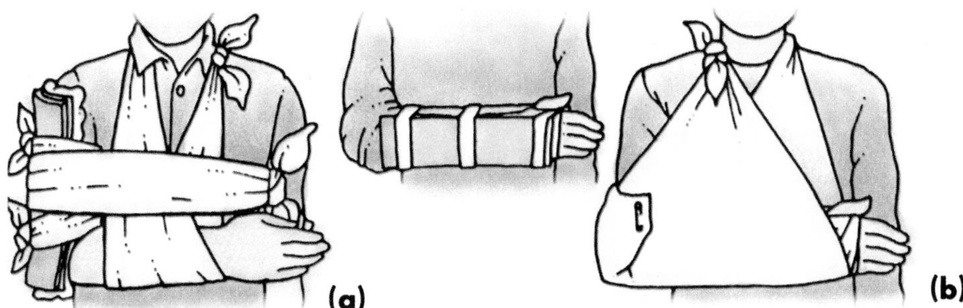

Methods of splinting: (a) arm in a sling, both strapped to the body; (b) splinted arm held in a sling.

tains injuries in a swimming pool, float him to the side and get adequate help before lifting him out of the water.

- While waiting for emergency help to arrive, check the pulse and respiration periodically, watch for shock, and keep the victim warm. Elevate his legs if signs of shock develop.

Skull fractures

A skull fracture, which could include brain injury, should be suspected if the victim has lacerations on the face or head, if he received a blow on the head, lost consciousness, is mentally confused or lethargic, has memory loss or speech disturbances, is paralyzed or convulses, or if the pupils are of unequal size. Another sign of skull fracture is blood or clear fluid trickling from the nose or ears.

First aid

- Treat the injury as though a neck fracture existed, since head and neck fractures may occur simultaneously.
- Check the pulse and respiration, and administer artificial respiration or CPR as needed.
- Control bleeding by placing a sterile gauze (or clean cloth pad) over the injury and applying appropriate pressure.
- Check for signs of shock. Do not give fluids.
- Do not move the victim. Seek professional help immediately.

Pelvic or hip fractures

These fractures occur from falls, especially in the elderly, and not infrequently happen spontaneously because of weakened bones (osteoporosis). Symptoms include pain in the low back, accentuated by movement of the leg, and pain in the hip, groin, and pubic area.

First aid

- Do not move the victim. Movement may cause injury to the pelvic organs.

- If it becomes necessary to move the victim, use the same method as for fractures of the back.
- While waiting for medical help to arrive, keep the victim as comfortable as possible, and watch for signs of shock.

Rib fractures

Rib fractures result from falls, car accidents, or banging into a sharp object. Should the broken end of a rib pierce the lung or heart, or the blood vessels within the chest are ruptured, the victim's life is threatened. When a rib pierces a lung, the lung may collapse, and red, frothy blood may be coughed up.

When many ribs on one side are fractured, that part of the chest wall loses its rigidity (**flail chest**). When the victim inhales, the injured area sinks in, inhibiting his ability to fill his lungs with air. When he exhales, the area bulges out. The victim also avoids breathing, and especially coughing, because of the severe pain these cause.

First aid

- Check the victim's pulse and respiration, and watch for signs of shock. Take any appropriate steps.
- Evaluate the victim's problems.

If pain is the principal symptom, or if the victim has a flail chest (see above), the chest should be stabilized with a firm-fitting binder (a broad bandage or a series of bandages) placed snugly around the chest (beginning below the armpits) so he can breathe more freely and the weakened area of the chest wall does not bulge with each exhalation.

- Place the victim in a slightly reclining position to make breathing easier.
- See your physician or go to a hospital emergency room.

Methods of splinting: (a) leg in a padded splint, made rigid with a stick; (b) leg splinted between two padded boards; (c) injured leg is splinted to the good leg.

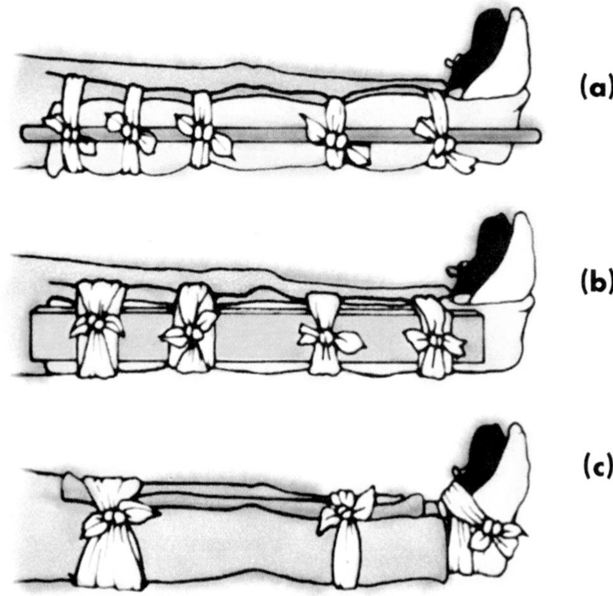

Wounds and injuries

A wound is an injury to the body in which the normal relationship of tissues is broken. If the break is in the covering tissues, such as the skin and mucous membranes, it is called an **open wound**. If it occurs in underlying tissues, it is spoken of as a **closed wound**.

There are a number of types of wounds: **abrasions**, in which the skin or membranes have been rubbed or scraped; **incisions**, in which the tissues have been cut with a knife or other sharp material such as glass or plastic; **lacerations**, in which the tissues have been torn apart by a blunt object, the edges being irregular; **punctures**, in which a hard object (a knife, bullet, nail, or thorn) makes a hole as it penetrates the skin or membrane and the underlying tissues; and **avulsions**, in which the tissues have been torn away from their supporting structures, such as loss of the scalp from hair being caught in a drill, or a leg lost in an explosion.

A wound is an injury to the body in which the normal relationship of tissues is broken.

Any part or organ of the body can sustain one or more of these wounds. Many of the specific injuries that the body experiences have already been described, and their care has been outlined.

Space does not permit a description of every type of injury to every organ and body structure. Here we will discuss the general principles of first-aid care for wounds and injuries that have not yet been described.

The first-aid care of wounds and injuries

- Do only that which preserves life, prevents further injury, and promotes healing.
- For any serious injury, call for trained medical help immediately, and when necessary, transport the victim to a physician, an emergency room, or a hospital.
- Keep the airway open, check for breathing and pulse, and when needed, administer artificial respiration or CPR (pages 6-9).
- Watch for shock, and give shock care if needed (page 10).
- Stop bleeding immediately. Place a sterile gauze or clean cloth pad over the lesion, and apply pressure. If this fails, apply pressure to the blood vessels supplying the area at suitable pressure points. If this is unsuccessful and the wound is on one of the limbs, apply a

tourniquet as a last resort.

- If the wound is on a limb and there is no fracture, elevate the limb to reduce bleeding.
- Do not try to clean the wound, except for irrigation with cool water to remove foreign bodies and to relieve pain. Cover the area with sterile gauze, a clean cloth, a piece of plastic, or even tinfoil.
- Immobilize the injured area.
- If the victim has sustained a back, neck, or head injury, do not move him except to save his life from a fire, explosion, drowning, etc., and then follow specific procedures.

Abdominal injuries

Injuries in which the abdomen has been torn open or received a stab or gunshot wound are gravely serious, as hemorrhage and infection may both occur.

First aid

- Keep the victim lying on his back. Place a pad under the knees to keep them bent and to relax the abdominal muscles.
- If the intestines protrude, do not try to replace them. Cover them with a clean cloth or a piece of plastic or tinfoil.
- Control bleeding with a pressure pad.

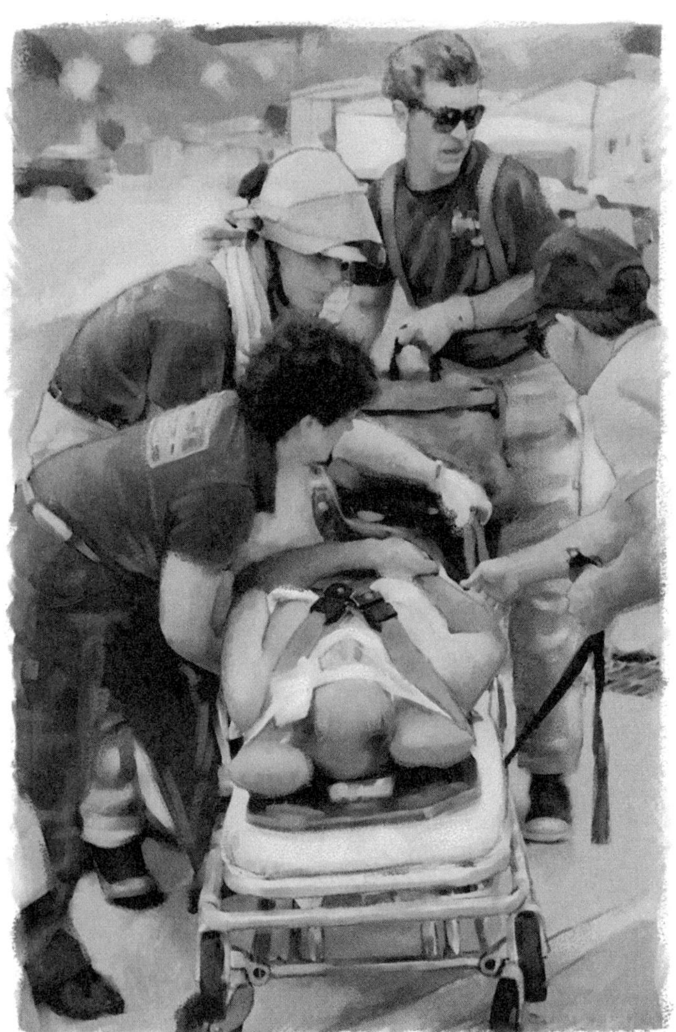

The immobilized victim is transported to the hospital.

Abrasions

Here the skin has been forcefully scuffed or scraped off. Frequently, small particles of dirt, sand, and other foreign material have been ground in.

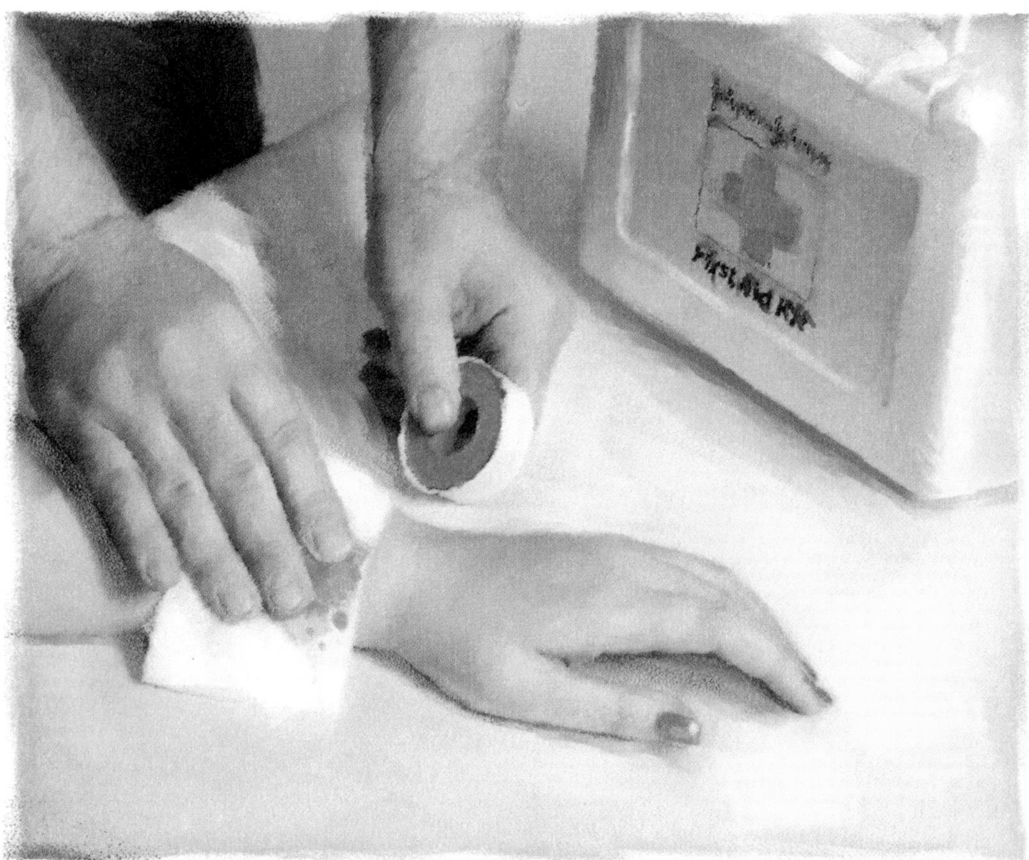

The edges of a superficial cut can be drawn together with adhesive tape or Band-Aids, and pressure applied till bleeding stops.

First aid

- Remove the clothing covering the injured area, and gently clean the wound with soap and water, removing as much of the dirt that has been ground in as possible. Cover the wound with a sterile gauze or clean cloth.
- Check with a physician about the advisability of a tetanus toxoid booster.

Bruises (contusions)

A bruise is an injury to tissues deep to (underneath) the skin in which the skin itself is usually not broken. Bruises are caused by a blow, falling against a hard object, or being struck by a solid object. The small blood vessels rupture and bleed into the tissues. Disintegrating blood causes the familiar "black and blue" discoloration that is evident as the lesion heals.

First aid

- Cold compresses during the first twenty-four hours tend to reduce swelling.

- Contrasting hot-and-cold applications thereafter increase circulation and promote healing.

Black eye

Treat as a bruise (contusion). If the victim has double vision, consult a physician.

Bruised fingertip (fingernail)

Fingertips are often caught in a door or smashed with a hammer. Blood often accumulates under the nail, and because of intense pressure from within, the pain is excruciating.

First aid

- Treat as a bruise (contusion).
- To relieve the intense pain from blood accumulating beneath the nail, heat a paper clip or wire (the thickness of a pencil lead) in a flame till it is red hot, then gently press the red-hot end on the nail above the accumulated blood. A hole will be formed and the blood released.

Penetrating chest wound

These are made by a knife, bullet, or any object that passes through the chest wall. Air can be sucked into the space around the lung, and the lung may collapse.

First aid

- Ask the victim to forcefully breathe out, and immediately apply a pressure dressing (gauze or pad of clean cloth) over the wound. Hold the dressing in place till professional help arrives, or, if such help is not immediately available, secure it with a snug bandage. Go to an emergency room.

Cuts and lacerations

Cuts are openings made in the skin or mucous membrane by a sharp instrument (knife, glass, metal, wood). Cuts open and bleed easily. Lacerations are tears caused by blunt objects that leave jagged edges.

First aid

- The edges of a superficial cut can be drawn together with adhesive tape or Band-Aids, and pressure applied till bleeding stops.
- For a cut that has passed through the deep layer of the skin and entered underlying tissues, suturing may be necessary. This is especially true of lacerations in which the edges may have to be trimmed. See a physician or go to an emergency room.

Sprains

Sprains are caused by a sudden and forceful twisting and wrenching of a joint, accompanied by stretching or tearing of the surrounding ligaments, tendons, muscles, and blood vessels. The ankles, fingers,

Ankles, fingers, wrists, and knees are the common areas for sprains.

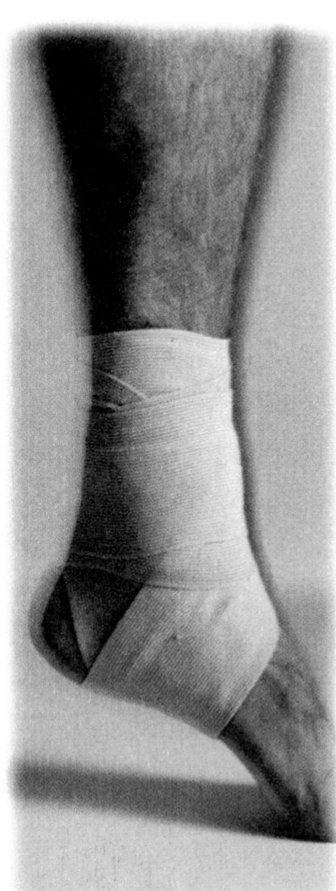

wrists, and knees are most frequently involved. The usual symptoms are immediate pain, especially when moving the affected part, with swelling and tenderness.

Strains result from overuse or overexertion of a muscle, which causes its fibers to stretch excessively and sometimes rupture.

First aid

- For a **mild sprain**, keep the injured part raised and apply cold or ice packs for the first day to reduce swelling.
- For a **severe sprain**, provide similar first aid as for a fracture, as one cannot be distinguished from the other. See a physician or go to an emergency room. An X-ray will determine the type of injury and the appropriate treatment. Severe sprains often require immobilization similar to fractures.
- Medication may be given for severe pain.

Strains

Strains result from overuse or overexertion of a muscle, which causes its fibers to stretch excessively and sometimes rupture. A strain may occur from improperly lifting a heavy weight, from athletic activities, from carrying a heavy suitcase without sufficient rest periods, or even from missing a step while descending a stairway.

First aid

- Treat **back strains** with bed rest on a very firm mattress and the application of heat. Should pain persist or the back strain be severe, consult a physician, as the problem may be a herniated disc.
- For strains of the arm or leg muscles, rest, together with warm, wet applications, should bring significant relief.
- Medication may be given for severe pain.

Environmental overexposure

Excessive exposure to cold, heat, or sun can cause serious damage to tissues of the body and may have life-threatening consequences if the whole body is involved. Body heat generated from intense exercise may have similar effects.

Frostbite (cold injury)

Frostbite is the actual freezing of the tissues of some part of the body, most often of the toes, fingers, ears, nose, or cheeks. Just before freezing, the skin appears violet-red, but changes to gray-yellow once it has frozen. A common sign of frostbite is gradual loss of pain, feeling, and function. Do not rub or massage the frozen parts with snow. This results in greater tissue loss.

First aid

- If the first aid is given out-of-doors, wrap the frozen part with a dry coat, blanket, or even several layers of newspaper.
- If help is rendered outside a hospital, in a house, warm the frozen area immediately by soaking it in warm water (101° to 105°F or 38° to 40°C). Do not use a heat lamp, hot water bottle, or heat from a stove. Warming may take up to an hour. The victim will experience pain, possibly severe, as the frozen tissue warms and as feeling and function return. Blisters may form, but should not be broken, and the area will swell severely.
- Elevate the affected part. Do not put pressure on it, but gently exercise it.
- Cover with a sterile bandage or clean cloth.
- Go immediately to an emergency room. Be careful not to allow refreezing, as this seriously damages the tissues. It is better to delay thawing if refreezing is possible.

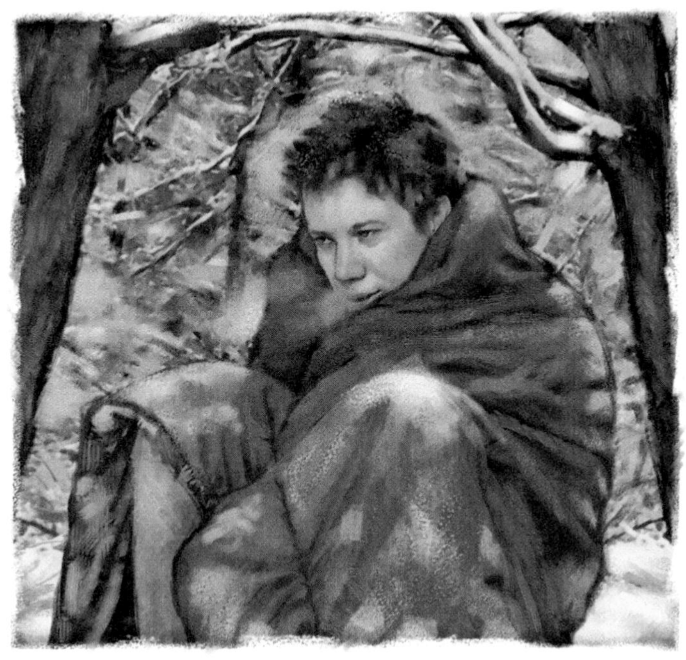

Frostbite is the actual freezing of the tissues of some part of the body, most often of the toes, fingers, ears, nose, or cheeks.

Hypothermia

Hypothermia refers to a condition in which the body temperature drops below normal (98.6°F or 37°C). When more body heat is lost than is replaced (as during prolonged exposure to very cold, windy conditions), body temperature gradually falls, and physical and mental functions slow down. The elderly, the very young, alcoholics, and persons taking psychotropic medications are most susceptible. The victim progressively exhibits shivering, numbness, stumbling, slurred speech, mental confusion, drowsiness, and coma, terminating in cardiac arrest and death.

First aid

- Check the victim's vital signs

Heat cramps, seen during intense exercise, are painful contractions of the muscle. Evidence suggests that dehydration is the cause.

and give artificial respiration if needed.

- Wrap the victim in blankets or warm clothes, and promptly take him to a shelter or emergency room. Hot-water bottles will provide additional heat, but do not use them in areas that may be frostbitten.
- Remove wet or damp clothes, and if the hypothermia is mild (the person is mentally alert but extremely cold), give a hot drink, **but NO alcohol**.
- If the hypothermia is severe, wrap the victim in warm blankets, or immerse him in a tub of water that is warm to the skin of the elbow. The water must not be hot. Rewarming may take several hours.
- Some victims go into shock during rewarming, and for that reason it is best if the rewarming can be done in a hospital or emergency room. If this is impossible (as on a camping trip), put the victim in a sleeping bag with a normally warm (euthermic) second person.

Heat cramps

Heat cramps, seen during intense exercise, are painful contractions of the muscles. It has long been held that the primary cause was salt depletion. Evidence now suggests that dehydration is the real cause and that salt depletion rarely occurs.

First aid

- Massage and gently stretch the cramped muscles. Contracting the opposing group of muscles appears to be quite effective.
- Have the victim drink lots of water. Salt should not be required unless the victim drinks more than 10 quarts (9 liters). Drinking generously before, during, and after strenuous exercise will generally prevent these painful cramps.

Heat exhaustion (heat prostration)

Heat exhaustion may develop from prolonged exposure to excessive heat and high humidity or from intense exercise (more commonly in a hot, humid environment), because the body's heat-dissipating mechanisms are inadequate to remove the heat being produced. The symptoms include a moderate rise in body temperature (102°F or 39°C), profuse sweating, clammy skin, fatigue, rapid breathing, headache, heat cramps, and the tendency to faint. Dehydration is common.

First aid

- Give plenty of water, and if the victim feels nauseated, have him sip the water.
- Take the victim to a cool environment. Place moist cloths on his forehead and wrists, and turn a fan on him if one is

available.

- Have the victim lie down and raise his feet a foot (30 cm) above the level of his head.
- If the victim is unconscious, take him to a hospital immediately. If the hospital is some distance away, give a retention enema of plain water, which will be absorbed.

Heatstroke (sunstroke)

Heatstroke is the most serious form of heat injury. Young people are most likely to experience heatstroke when undergoing strenuous exercise. However, elderly persons and those who are ill may develop heatstroke without active exercise. The precipitating cause is high environmental temperature and humidity. The symptoms, which come on abruptly, include flushed, hot, dry skin; no sweating; mental confusion; lethargy; and rapid onset of coma. Body temperature may rise to 106°F (41°C) or higher. If treatment is not instituted immediately, the victim will go into shock. The higher the body temperature, the worse the prognosis.

First aid

- Heatstroke is a medical emergency. Take the victim to the nearest hospital or emergency room. When this is not possible, the following will be helpful.
- Cool the victim to lower his body temperature. Placing the victim in a tub of ice-cold water has long been recommended. This, however, tends to induce shivering, which, in turn, raises the body's core temperature. Better results have been obtained by continuously sponging the face, body, and limbs with cool water. A fan blowing on the victim will aid cooling. Reduce the cooling measures when the body temperature has fallen to 102°F (39°C) to keep the victim's temperature from dropping too low.
- If the victim is in a hospital, fluids can be given intravenously. When this is not possible and

Heatstroke is the most serious form of heat injury.

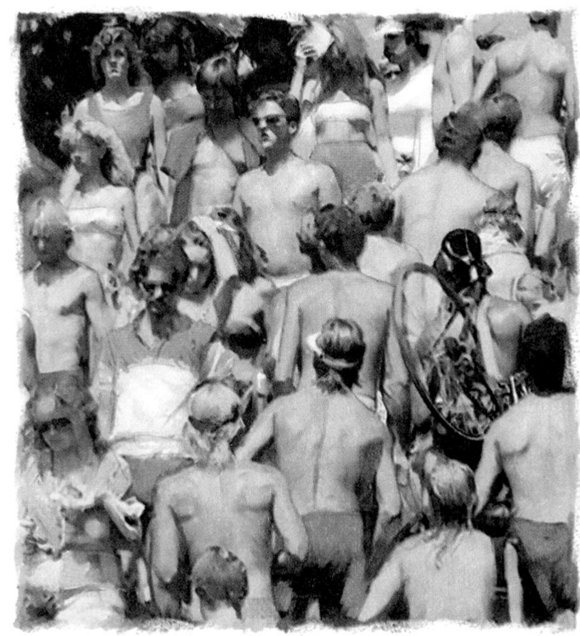

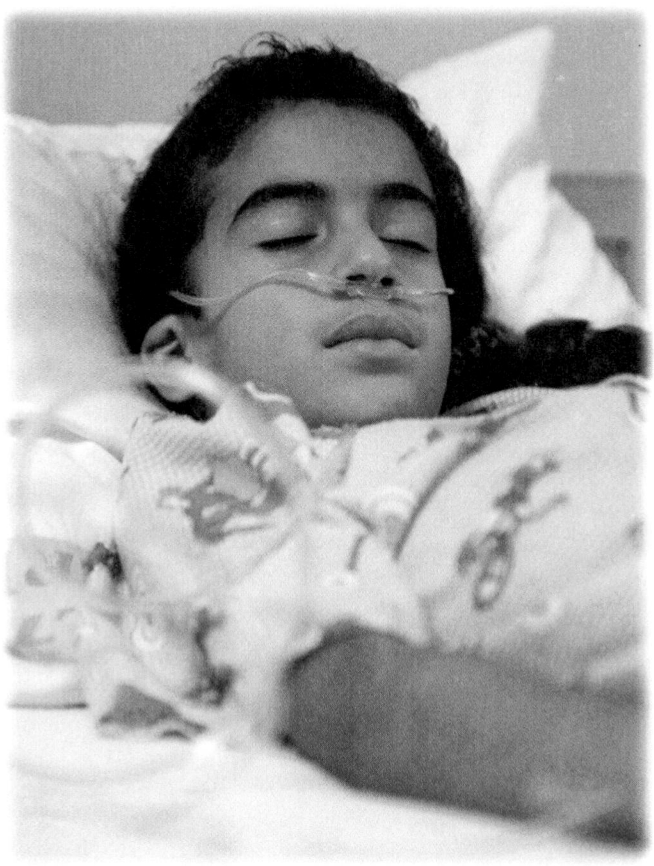

A few of the more common causes of unconsciousness include head injuries, poisoning, drug overdoses, and cardiac arrests.

the victim is conscious, have him drink a glass of water (8 oz or 250 ml) every twenty minutes.

- When the body temperature has reached normal, dry the victim off. However, check his body temperature for a while, and if it starts to rise again, resume cooling measures.
- **Do NOT give alcoholic beverages.**

Unconsciousness (coma)

A number of conditions may cause unconsciousness. A few of the more common ones include heart attack, stroke, diabetic coma (too little insulin and too much blood sugar), hypoglycemia (too much insulin and too little blood sugar), a head injury, uremia, poisoning, or a drug overdose, and cardiac arrest.

First aid

- In all cases, summon medical help or take the victim to an emergency room.
- In the meantime, keep him warm, keep his airway open, and, should breathing cease, give artificial respiration. If the heart stops, start CPR.

Fainting

Fainting is a temporary loss of consciousness due to a reduction of blood flowing to the brain. A common cause is emotional concern although fainting may have a variety of causes.

First aid

- Have the victim lie on the floor and elevate his feet. Consciousness will usually be regained quickly. If it does not return within one or two minutes, call a physician.
- If a person is about to faint, have him sit down and lean forward, putting his head between

his knees. Then have him try to raise his head while someone else is pushing his head downward. This will force blood to the brain, which should prevent fainting.

Convulsions

A convulsion is a sudden onset of unconsciousness accompanied by rigidity, followed by jerky contractions of the body muscles (**seizure**). While the muscles are rigid, the victim stops breathing, loses control of his bladder and bowel, and may bite his tongue. The many causes of convulsions include **epilepsy**, head injury, stroke, meningitis, withdrawal from alcohol or drugs, drug overdose, poisonings, and, in children, high fever.

First aid

- Protect the victim against injury. Lay him down on a soft surface if one is available. Place a rolled-up handkerchief between his upper and lower jaws (teeth), **not** a hard, blunt object.
- Allow the victim to convulse. Do **not** restrain his movements.
- Do **not** put a child with a high fever in a tub of water, but sponge him down with lukewarm water.
- Do not try to give fluids, but provide artificial respiration or CPR if needed (pages 6-9).
- Following the seizure, allow the victim to sleep and rest.
- Seek medical help.

Delirium

Delirium is a state of mental haziness ("out of his head") in which the victim is confused, restless, anxious, and unable to cooperate, and his imagination is out of control. Causes include high fever, acute intoxication with alcohol or other drugs, poisonings, and many serious illnesses.

Fainting is a temporary loss of consciousness due to a reduction of blood flowing to the brain.

First aid

- Protect the victim from injury and keep him in a quiet environment.
- Seek medical help. If this is delayed and the victim can cooperate, encourage him to drink water.

Drowning and near-drowning

Drowning occurs when water enters the voice box (larynx), which then goes into spasm, or when water floods the lungs (air passageways). If he is not rescued within minutes, the victim will sustain permanent damage to his brain and

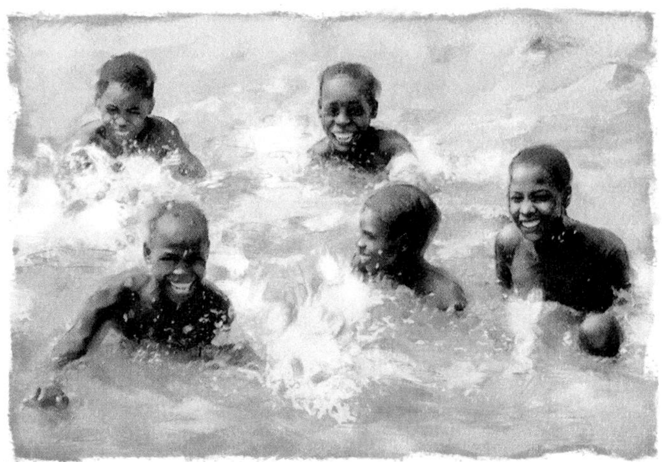

Drowning is a serious concern of water-related recreational sports.

other organs from a lack of oxygen. If he is deprived of oxygen too long, he will die.

Drownings are America's fourth leading cause of accidental deaths, the highest drowning rate being among infants less than one year of age. Of these, some 70 percent drown in the bathtub. A growing number of children die in outdoor hot tubs. Fifty percent of drownings among youth and adults are related to the use of alcohol. Drowning is a serious concern of water-related recreational sports.

Drownings are America's fourth leading cause of accidental deaths.

The steps in drowning may vary, but they commonly follow this sequence: the victim panics, and while struggling to stay above water, breathes rapidly and deeply. He then becomes exhausted and holds his breath as his head goes down. He swallows water, vomits, and then coughs violently. Eventually he gasps, and his lungs fill with water. This is followed by unconsciousness, convulsions, and death.

Cautions

- Unless he is trained and capable of assisting a drowning person, an inexperienced observer should not jump into the water to save the victim, but should **summon help**. Far too many would-be rescuers have drowned with their drowning victims.
- Throw the victim a life jacket, a plastic bottle, a rope-anything that will float or that he can grasp onto while being pulled to shore.
- If a boat is available, row out to the victim and tow him to shore. Do not try to pull the victim aboard, as the boat may capsize.
- If the incident resulted from a water accident that may have caused neck or back injuries, do not lift the victim directly out of the water. Float him to shore, or place a board or stretcher underneath him and then lift him out of the water.
- If the victim has fallen through thin ice, have him place his arms and chest on the edge of

the ice, then throw him a rope or extend a long board to him and pull him onto the ice. If enough rescuers are available, have them lie face down on the ice and form a human chain out to the victim.

First aid

- If the victim's breathing has stopped, give mouth-to-mouth respiration, if possible while he is still in the water. If his chest does not inflate, do not drain water from his lungs, but blow more forcibly into his lungs. Take special precaution not to overinflate the lungs of an infant or small child.
- Once the victim is on shore, if he has no pulse, start CPR (page 8). Continue for one hour unless he revives sooner. Take him to a hospital immediately, as serious complications may develop following a near-drowning.

Diving emergencies

Diving. Serious injuries to the head and neck may result from diving and striking one's head against a rock or the floor of a swimming pool.

Deep diving. With scuba-diving equipment, swimmers can dive to depths of more than 100 feet (30 m). Drowning can result from failure of equipment to provide air or oxygen and from the lines becoming entangled in weeds or rocks.

Decompression sickness, "the bends." Divers who remain too long at depths greater than 30 feet (10 m) and then ascend to the surface without allowing enough time for the gases dissolved in the blood and body fluids to reach a new equilibrium (decompression) develop

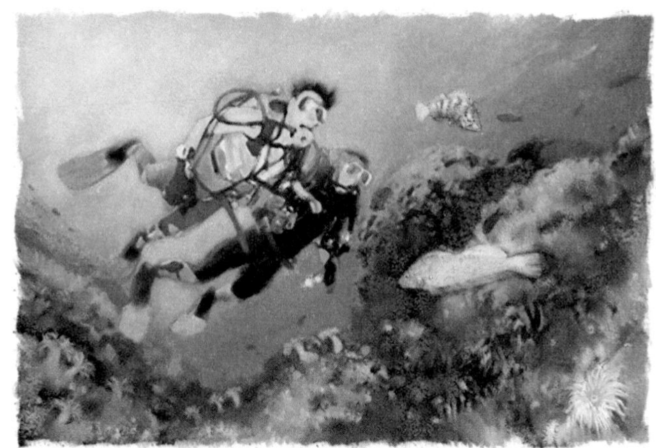

gas bubbles in their tissues, with serious aftereffects.

Symptoms occurring soon after emerging from the water include pain in the joints, pain in the chest with cough and difficult breathing, paralysis of certain muscles, disturbances of vision, and dizziness.

First aid

- For striking one's head when **diving**, see "neck fracture," page 51.
- For **drowning or near-drowning** when deep diving, see

Serious injuries to the head and neck may result from diving and striking one's head against a rock or the floor of a swimming pool.

"drowning," page 63.

- For **decompression sickness**, special pressure equipment is required. Ask official lifeguards where such equipment is available and call for professional help. If the help is delayed very long, the victim, if physically able, may dive to depths that will redissolve the gas bubbles and then ascend more deliberately.

Far too many would-be rescuers have drowned with their drowning victims.

Hernia

A hernia is a protrusion of the bowel through a weakness in the abdominal wall.

First aid

- It is usually simple, especially to begin with, to push a hernia back into the abdomen (reduce) by applying pressure on the protrusion with the fingers. Having the victim lie on his back, with his hips slightly elevated and his knees drawn up to his shoulders, will aid in the procedure. If this is unsuccessful, have the victim consult a physician immediately.

Hiccup

A hiccup is a sudden, uncontrolled, fitful contraction of the diaphragm, during which inhalation is abruptly stopped by closure of the larynx. Hiccups usually occur at intervals of a few seconds, and most attacks end in a few minutes. Sometimes, however, especially following abdominal surgery or in connection with serious illnesses, an attack may last hours or even days, and become life threatening.

First aid

- A number of simple, harmless procedures are advocated to end a hiccup: drinking water; while stooping forward, drinking water from the side of the glass away from you; holding your breath; sucking ice; and breathing into a paper sack held over your nose and mouth.
- If these simple measures are ineffective, see a physician.

Alcoholic intoxication

An individual's capacity to function physically and mentally is impaired when he is intoxicated with alcohol. He is sluggish, uncoordinated, and clumsy. He is mentally dull, his judgment is faulty, and his understanding is distorted. At times he may be violent, and he can be dangerous. Or he may go into a stupor and lapse into a coma.

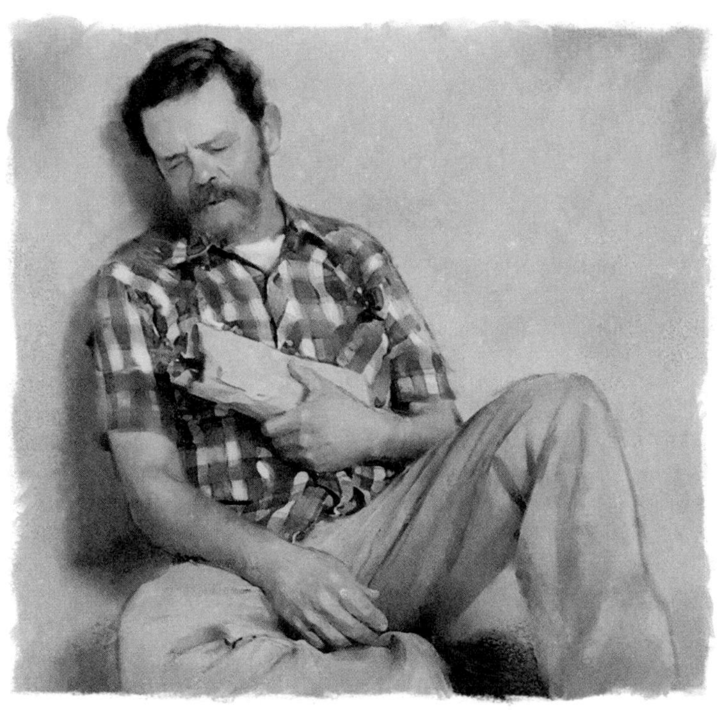

First aid

- Should the intoxicated person show signs of shock (cold, clammy skin; rapid, weak pulse; and irregular breathing), seek professional medical help.
- If the victim's breathing becomes inhibited, give him artificial respiration (page 6). Keep his airway open, turning his head to one side so that vomitus will flow out of his mouth.
- Keep the victim warm. Intoxicated persons lose heat more rapidly than normal individuals.

Vomiting

Vomiting may be due to dietary indiscretion or a temporary gastrointestinal infection, or it may indicate a serious illness. If simple measures do not relieve the problem within a day, see a physician.

First aid

- Put the victim to bed and keep him warm.
- Encourage him to drink plenty of fluids. Give him sips of ice-cold water or have him suck ice or give him hot, clear broth to drink, again in sips.
- If vomiting continues, call a physician, who will determine the underlying cause and may prescribe an antivomiting medication.
- If the victim is unconscious, keep his airway clear of the vomitus and get medical help.

An individual's capacity to function physically and mentally is impaired when he is intoxicated with alcohol.

The home medicine chest and first-aid kits

- Precautions
- Contents of a medicine chest
- Common uses of medications
- First-aid kits

Surveys have shown that nine out of ten aches and pains, together with minor injuries, are brushed off or treated by the sufferer with some readily available medication or simple procedure. Of the remaining problems, less than half are cared for by trained health professionals. The home medicine chest is usually a ready source of band-aids and bandages, ointments, disinfectants, and remedies for headaches, upset stomachs, colds, coughs, diarrhea, and constipation.

Precautions

The most important rule for your medicine cabinet is "Be careful!" Parents and guardians of small children should be aware that aspirin and iron are among the most common forms of poisoning among children. Children like to play doctor and nurse, and when parents are not watching, they sometimes frequent the medicine cabinet. The result is often tragic. Medicines should be kept away from little hands, even when secured in child-resistant bottles. Children should be taught from babyhood never to take medicine unless a parent, nurse, or teacher gives it to them. Do not encourage a child to take a medicine by telling him that it's "candy." It may taste sweet, but it is not candy.

Note the expiration date of all medications that you purchase, whether with a prescription or over the counter. If you are in doubt about a medicine that has been

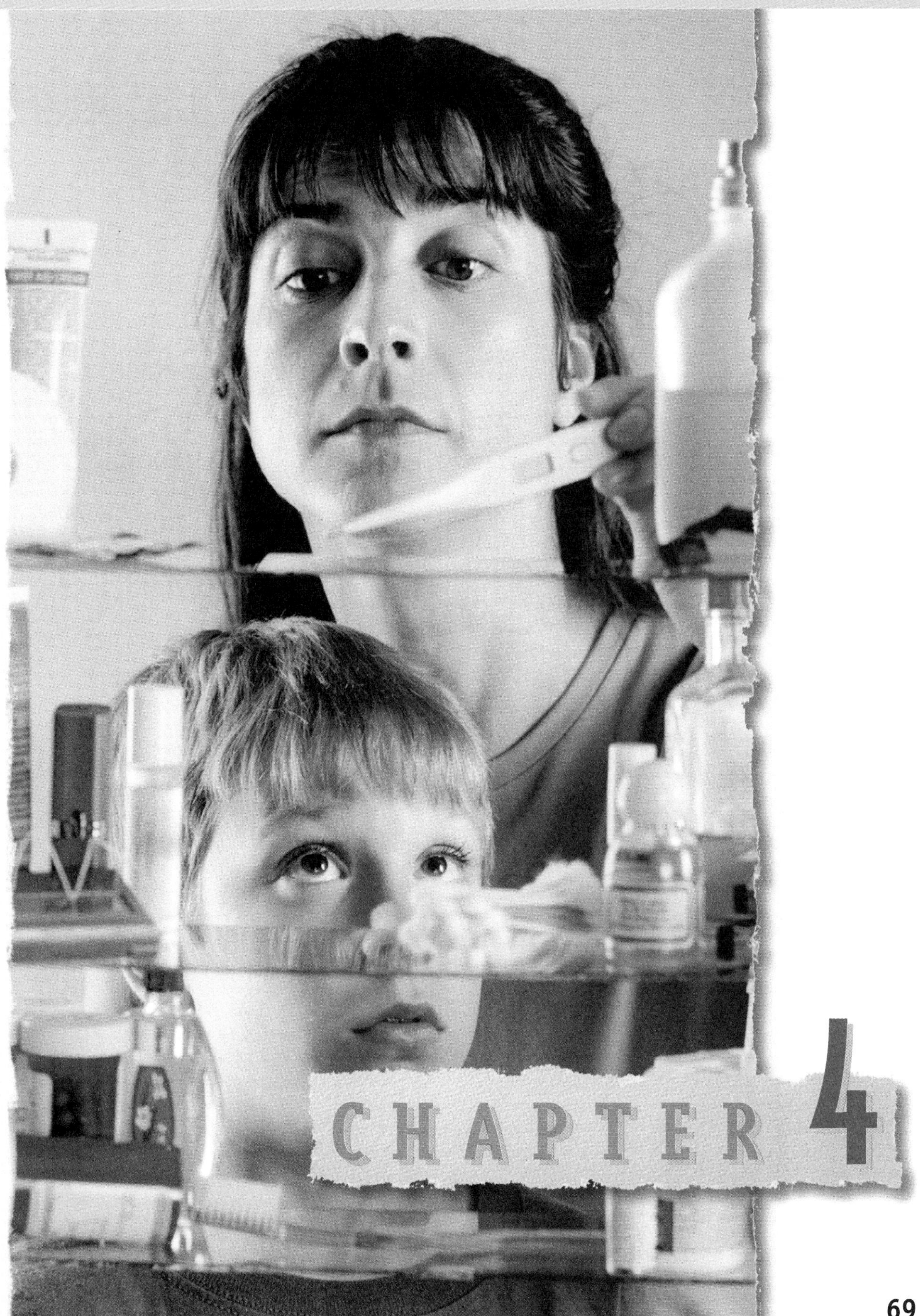

CHAPTER 4

around for a while, check with your pharmacist before using it. Your pharmacist can advise you as to which medicines should be stored in the refrigerator and which will keep well in a drawer or cupboard. All medicines should be labeled. *Never use medicine from a container that has no label.* Medicines should be kept out of reach of children or in a locked container or cupboard.

It is unwise to prescribe leftover medicines for another member of the family, or for a neighbor who appears to have the same problem you or someone in your family had. Before retaking a medication, check with your physician.

Do not discard tablets, capsules, injectables, or ointments in places where children may find them. Wherever possible, flush old medicines down the toilet. Otherwise, seal them in a childproof container and place them in the garbage. Always break off the needles on disposable syringes before throwing them away.

Contents of a medicine chest

It is important to stock your medicine cabinet ahead of time with certain basic items so that in a time of emergency you won't have to waste precious time going to the store to purchase what you need. The following list should be adequate as a start. You will, of course, add to it as time goes on. But always be sure you have an adequate supply of these items on hand:

Equipment

Scissors, medium size.
Medicine droppers, two.
Tweezers, sharp, pointed.
Rubber syringe, soft, small.
Disposable syringes with needles (1 ml), five.
Sewing needle, medium size.
Teaspoon or measuring cup, small.
Hot-water bottle.
Safety pins, six medium, six large.
Ice bag.
Razor blades, stiff-backed.
Clinical thermometers
- oral—one.
- rectal—one.

Flashlight.
Safety matches.

Supplies

Absorbent cotton, sterile, small roll.
Cotton balls, sterile, small bag.
Sterile gauze pads, prepackaged.
- four 2 inches (5 cm) square.
- four 4 inches (20 cm) square.

Cotton tip applicators—small package.
Adhesive tape, one roll, 1-inch (2.5 cm) wide.
Band-aids, one box, assorted sizes.
Roller bandages, gauze
- one roll, 1 inch (2.5 cm) wide.
- one roll, 2 inch (5 cm) wide.

Ace bandage, one 3 inch (7.5 cm) wide.
Enema kit (chemical)—one.
Rubbing alcohol, 16 ounce (500 ml), one bottle.
Baby oil, small bottle.
Petrolatum (Vaseline), 4 oz (100 gm).
Glycerin—8 oz (200 ml).
Activated charcoal—
- powder, 4 oz (100 gm)
- tablets, bottle of fifty.

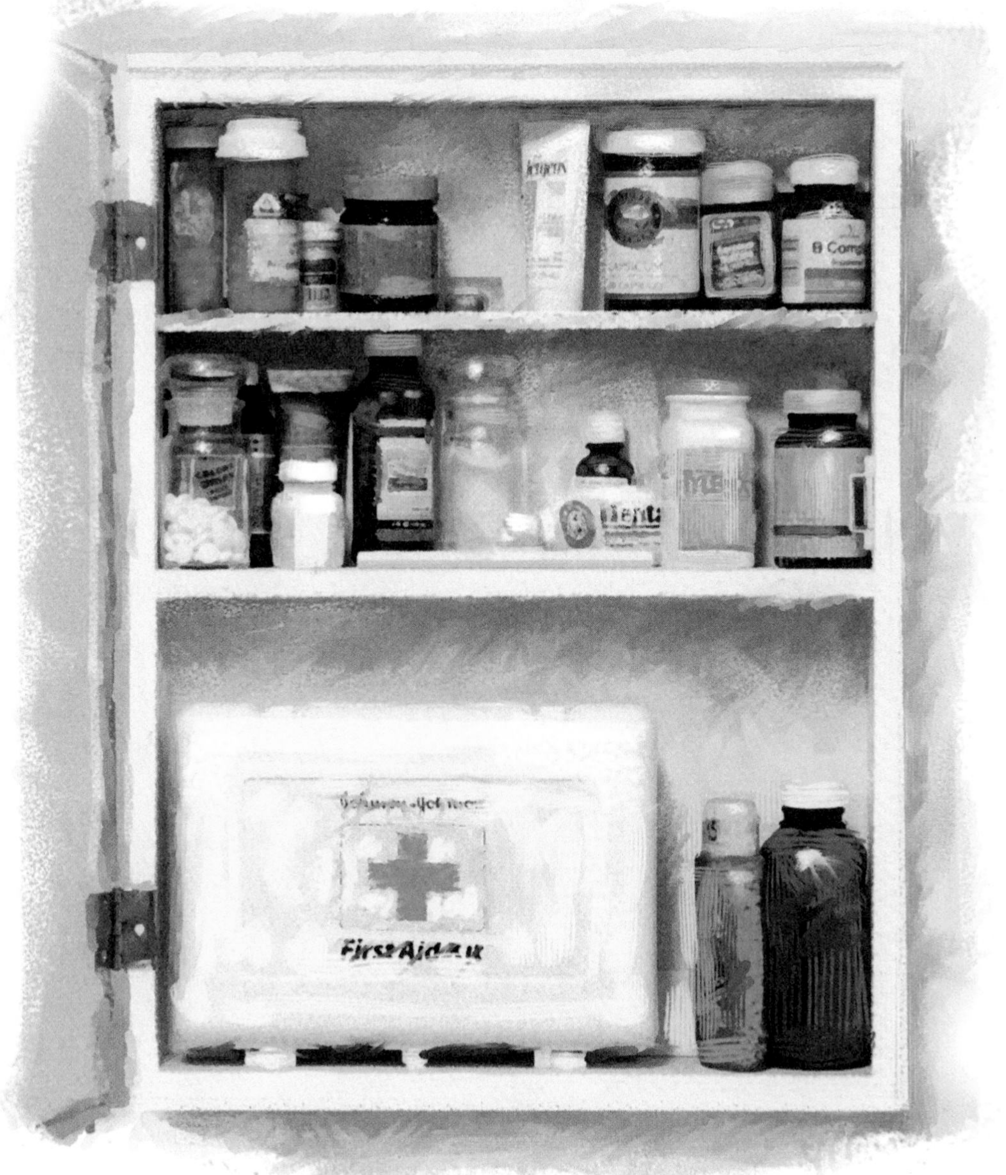

Antiseptic soap, bar or liquid.
Antiseptic, small bottle (for skin).
Milk of magnesia, medium bottle.

Medications

Boric acid ointment, 5 percent.
Zinc oxide ointment, small tube.
Eyewash, small bottle with eyecup.
Eucalyptus oil, small bottle.
Antihistamine, Chlor-Trimeton, twenty-five tablets.
Nitroglycerin, sublingual 0.3 mg, ten tablets.
Adrenalin (norepinephrine), injection five 1-ml vials with five 1-ml disposable syringes.
Milk of magnesia, medium bottle.
Epsom salts, 1 lb (500 mg).
Syrup of ipecac, 2 oz (50 ml).
Earache drops, small bottle.
Calamine lotion, 4 oz (100 ml).
Antacids, aluminum or magnesium hydroxide, twenty-five tablets.
Cough syrup, small bottle.
Tylenol, 120 mg, ten tablets.

Do not discard tablets, capsules, injectables, or ointments in places where children may find them.

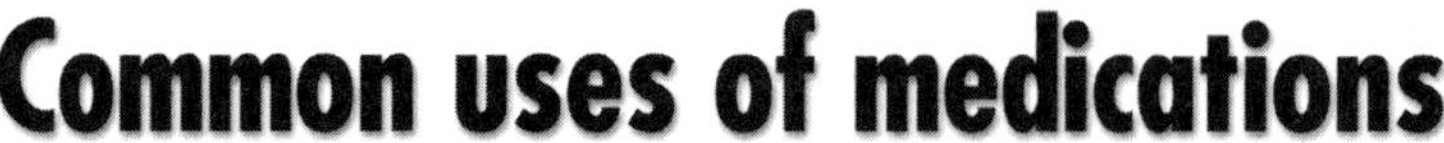

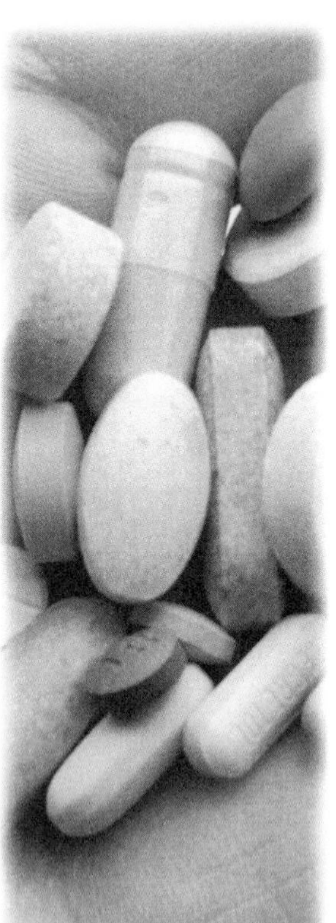

Glycerin: moisten lips or around mouth.

Charcoal: powder for poisonings; tablets for indigestion.

Boric acid ointment: prevents infection.

Zinc ointment: skin-drying effect, prevents infection.

Eucalyptus oil: for vaporizer.

Antihistamines: hay fever, sensitivity reaction.

Nitroglycerin: angina chest pain.
Adrenalin: for sensitivity to insect bite or sting.

Milk of magnesia: milk laxative.

Epsom salts: for catharsis, or arm or leg bath.

Syrup of ipecac: for controlled vomiting.

Ear drops: mild outer-ear infection.

Calamine lotion: for itching skin rash.

Antacids: occasional indigestion.

Cough syrup: for nonproductive cough.

Tylenol: mild muscle pains or transient headache.

Medicines for emergency use

Antiseptics: For any superficial wound that may become infected. It is perhaps more important to thoroughly cleanse the lesion with mild soap and water.

Emetics: These agents produce vomiting. Syrup of ipecac, when used, produces prompt vomiting. To induce vomiting, use Procedure 5, page 21.

Nitroglycerin: This medicine is most commonly used for relief of an angina attack.

Adrenalin: To be injected only in the event of a severe allergic reaction or anaphylactic shock. See page 35.

Antihistamine: Given in conjunction with adrenalin for a severe allergic reaction, or in case of stings of certain insects.

First-aid kits

Various manufacturers put together special first-aid packages or kits, often of sizes and shapes that are convenient for packing into a case. These kits are also packaged to prevent contamination or spoilage, and generally have printed directions for use on the outside. The extra cost of obtaining your first-aid kit in such form will probably repay you in the long run. Your pharmacist will doubtless be able to show you samples.

It would obviously be impossible to take along your entire medicine cabinet on a trip away from home. However, it is wise to take along those first-aid articles that you feel might be needed. If you are going into a country where poisonous snakes abound, be sure to add to your arsenal a snakebite kit (available commercially). If you have in your party someone who might suffer an angina attack, nitroglycerin tablets would be a wise choice. You might wish to prepare your own first-aid supplies and carry them in a small toolbox or a fisherman's tackle box.

Every family should have available for immediate use a book put out by the American Red Cross on first aid. This book presents very concisely what should be done under a large variety of emergency situations. The book is available at many bookstores and at the American Red Cross office nearest you.

Ready diagnosis of common problems

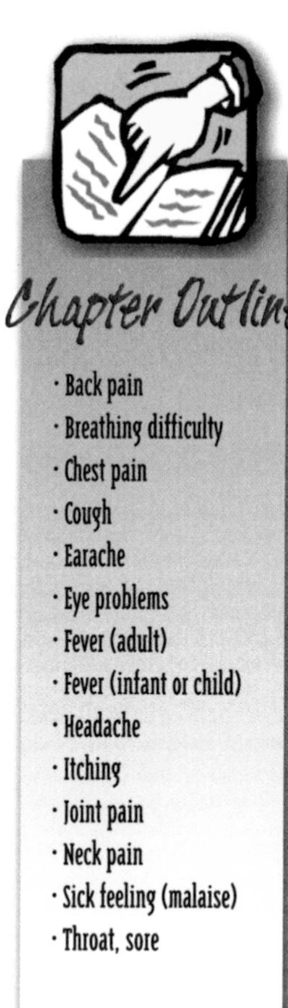
Chapter Outline
· Back pain
· Breathing difficulty
· Chest pain
· Cough
· Earache
· Eye problems
· Fever (adult)
· Fever (infant or child)
· Headache
· Itching
· Joint pain
· Neck pain
· Sick feeling (malaise)
· Throat, sore

The flowcharts on the pages that follow will help you to quickly diagnose some of the more common symptoms that people complain about. All of the questions can be answered by Yes or No. After you have answered a question, follow its answer to the next question and the next, till you reach the "end of the line," at which point recommendations will be made for treatment. You will be advised if you should consult a physician. Where the symptom suggests a medical emergency if it is not treated immediately, the box around the recommendation will be red.

The following example shows how to use these flowcharts. If your back pain is severe, you would answer Yes and follow the line to the box that asks, "Did it come on suddenly?" The bold lines are one possible series of answers that might be given, ending in the recommendation to "consult your physician immediately." Since this is a medical emergency, the box around this recommendation is printed in red.

Back pain

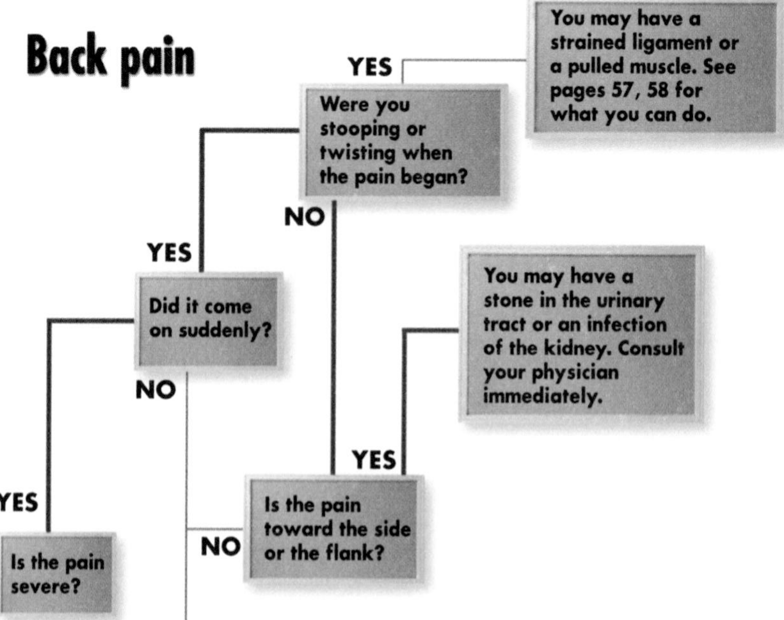
Is the pain severe?
YES
Did it come on suddenly?
YES
Were you stooping or twisting when the pain began?
YES
You may have a strained ligament or a pulled muscle. See pages 57, 58 for what you can do.
NO
Is the pain toward the side or the flank?
YES
You may have a stone in the urinary tract or an infection of the kidney. Consult your physician immediately.
NO
NO

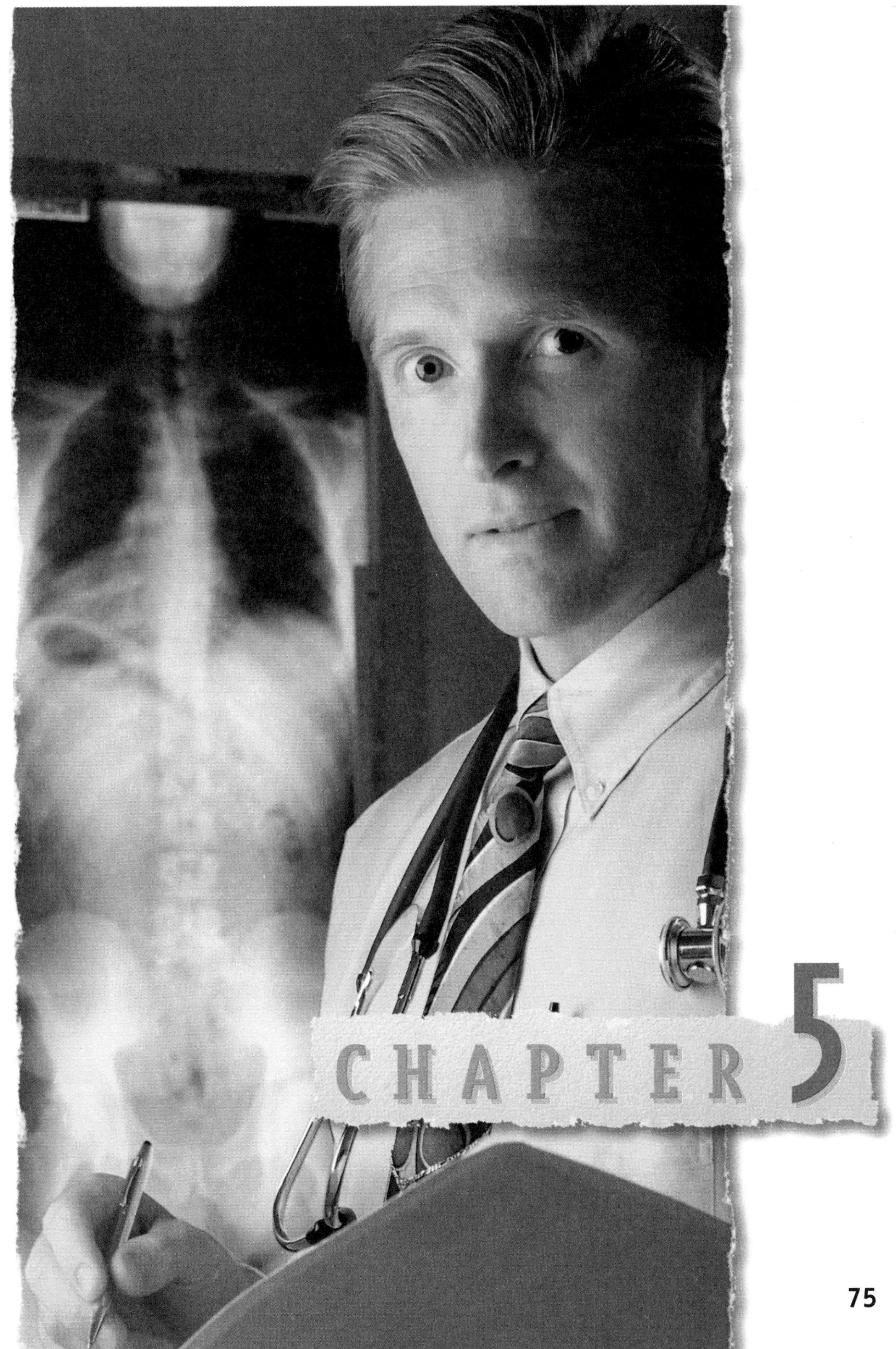

CHAPTER 5

Back pain

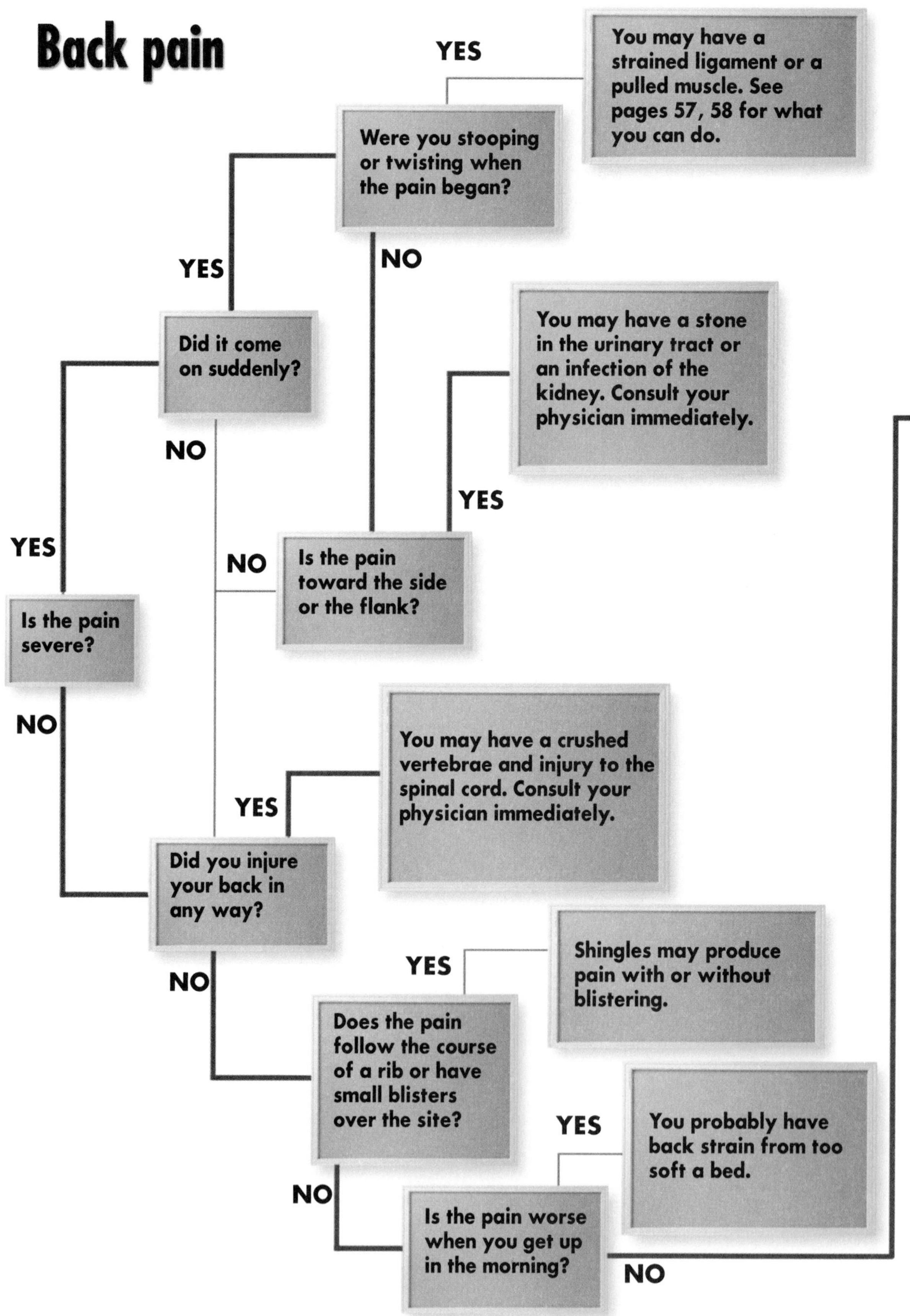

YES
You may have a strained ligament or a pulled muscle. See pages 57, 58 for what you can do.
Were you stooping or twisting when the pain began?
YES
NO
Did it come on suddenly?
You may have a stone in the urinary tract or an infection of the kidney. Consult your physician immediately.
NO
YES
YES
NO
Is the pain toward the side or the flank?
Is the pain severe?
NO
You may have a crushed vertebrae and injury to the spinal cord. Consult your physician immediately.
YES
Did you injure your back in any way?
Shingles may produce pain with or without blistering.
NO
YES
Does the pain follow the course of a rib or have small blisters over the site?
YES
You probably have back strain from too soft a bed.
NO
Is the pain worse when you get up in the morning?
NO

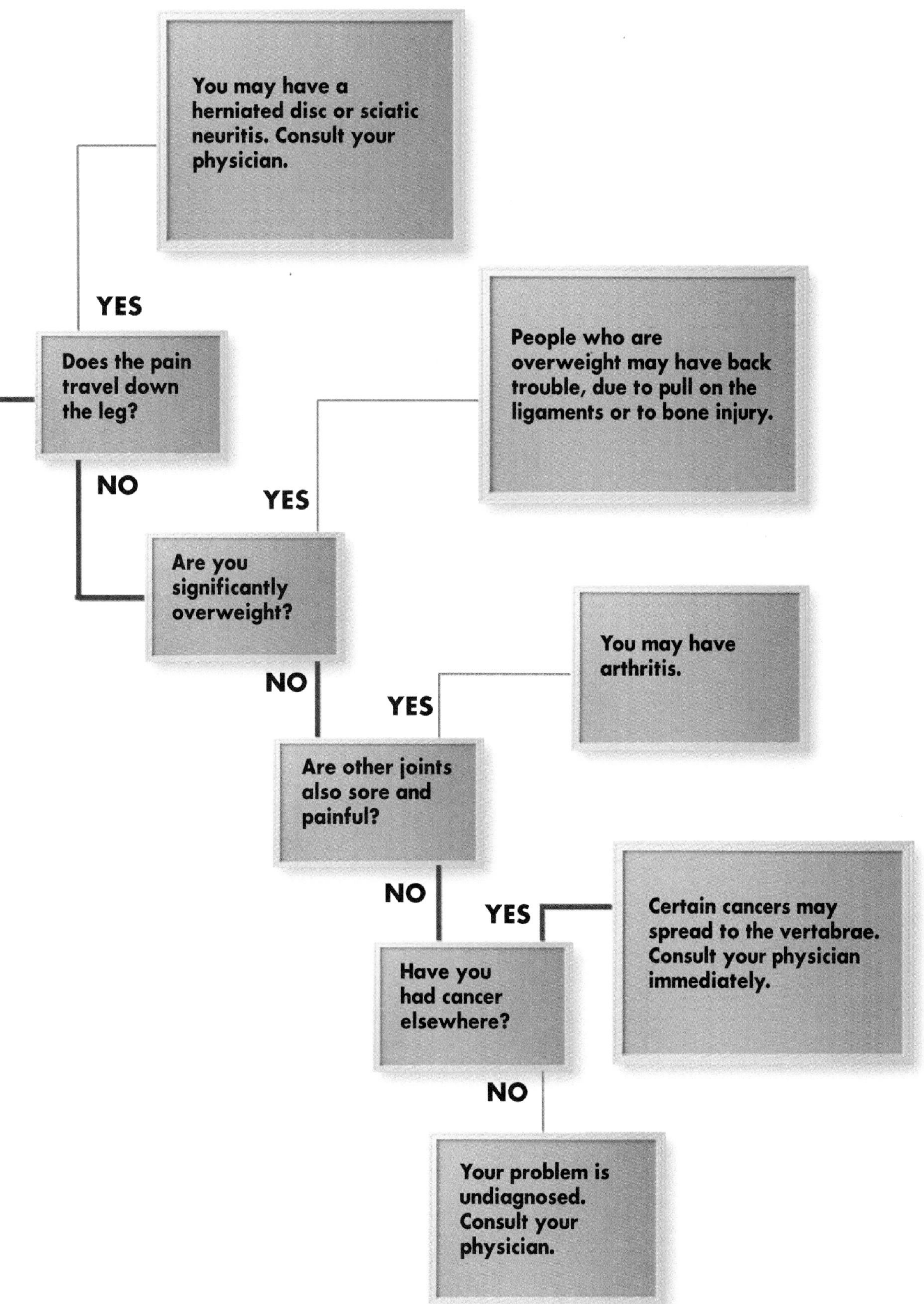
You may have a herniated disc or sciatic neuritis. Consult your physician.
YES
Does the pain travel down the leg?
NO
People who are overweight may have back trouble, due to pull on the ligaments or to bone injury.
YES
Are you significantly overweight?
NO
You may have arthritis.
YES
Are other joints also sore and painful?
NO
YES
Certain cancers may spread to the vertabrae. Consult your physician immediately.
Have you had cancer elsewhere?
NO
Your problem is undiagnosed. Consult your physician.

Breathing difficulty

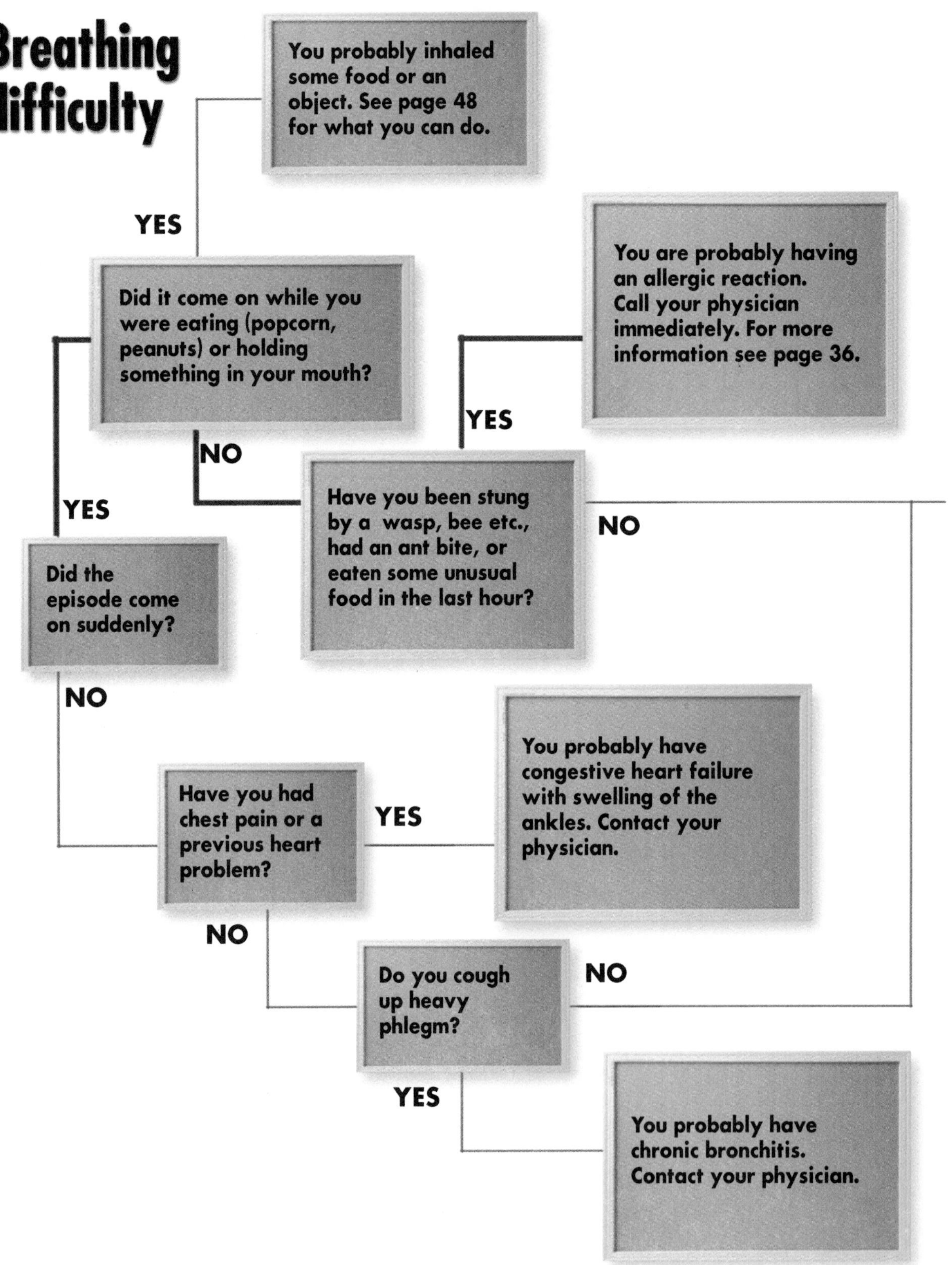

You probably inhaled some food or an object. See page 48 for what you can do.
YES
Did it come on while you were eating (popcorn, peanuts) or holding something in your mouth?
You are probably having an allergic reaction. Call your physician immediately. For more information see page 36.
YES
NO
Have you been stung by a wasp, bee etc., had an ant bite, or eaten some unusual food in the last hour?
NO
YES
Did the episode come on suddenly?
NO
You probably have congestive heart failure with swelling of the ankles. Contact your physician.
Have you had chest pain or a previous heart problem?
YES
NO
Do you cough up heavy phlegm?
NO
YES
You probably have chronic bronchitis. Contact your physician.

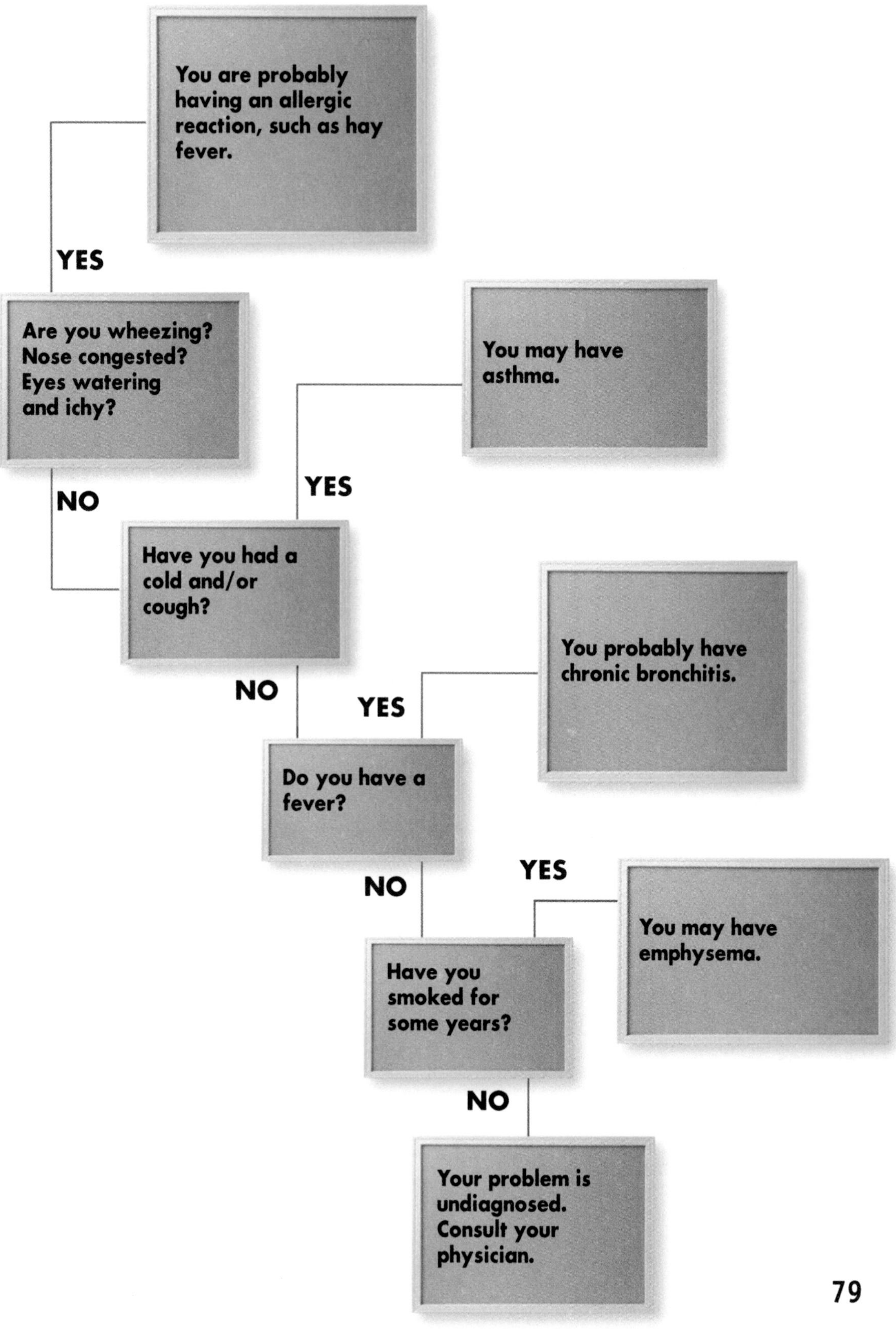
You are probably having an allergic reaction, such as hay fever.
YES
Are you wheezing? Nose congested? Eyes watering and ichy?
You may have asthma.
NO
YES
Have you had a cold and/or cough?
You probably have chronic bronchitis.
NO
YES
Do you have a fever?
YES
NO
You may have emphysema.
Have you smoked for some years?
NO
Your problem is undiagnosed. Consult your physician.

Chest pain

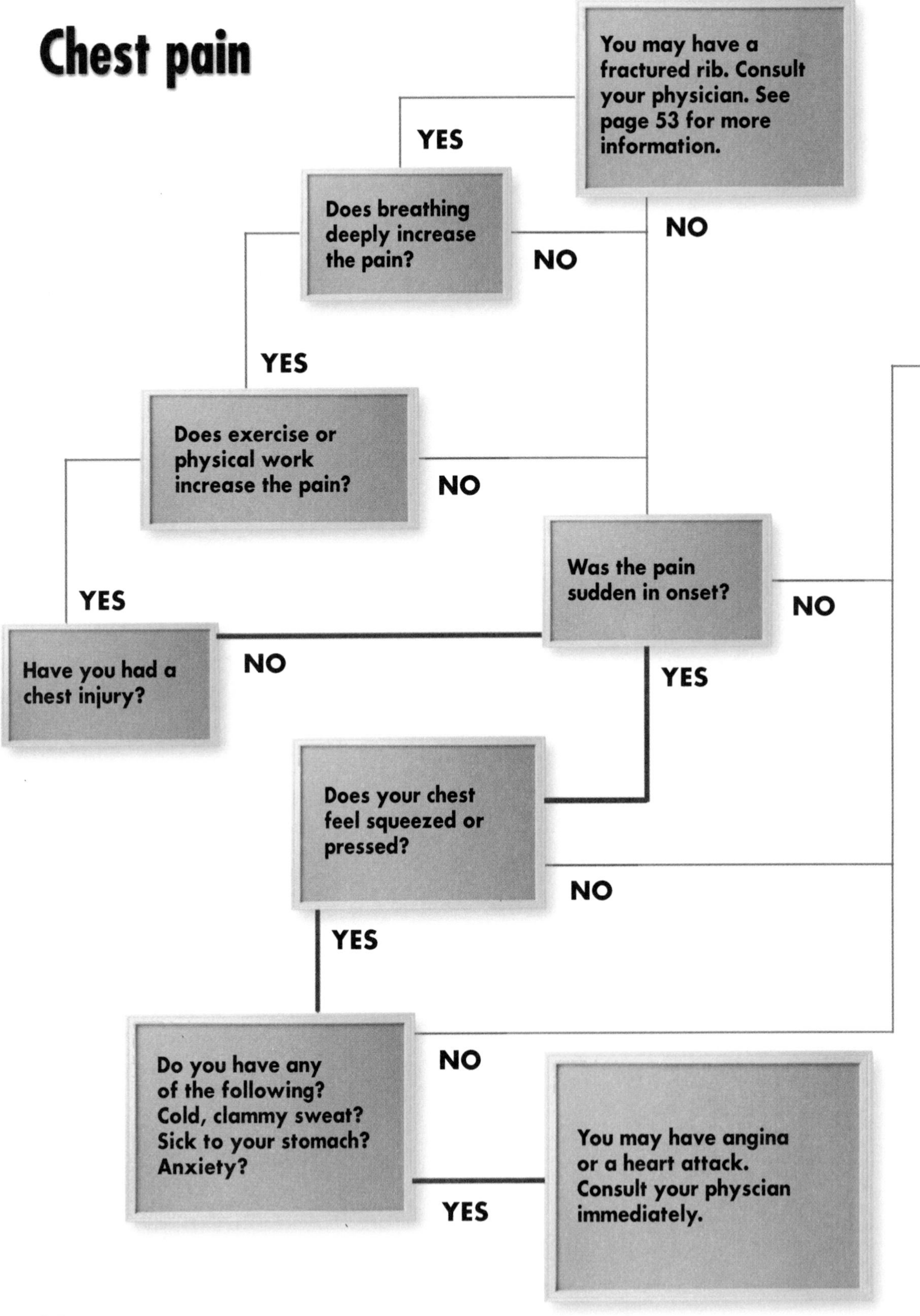

You may have a fractured rib. Consult your physician. See page 53 for more information.
YES
Does breathing deeply increase the pain?
NO
NO
YES
Does exercise or physical work increase the pain?
NO
Was the pain sudden in onset?
YES
NO
Have you had a chest injury?
NO
YES
Does your chest feel squeezed or pressed?
NO
YES
Do you have any of the following? Cold, clammy sweat? Sick to your stomach? Anxiety?
NO
YES
You may have angina or a heart attack. Consult your physcian immediately.

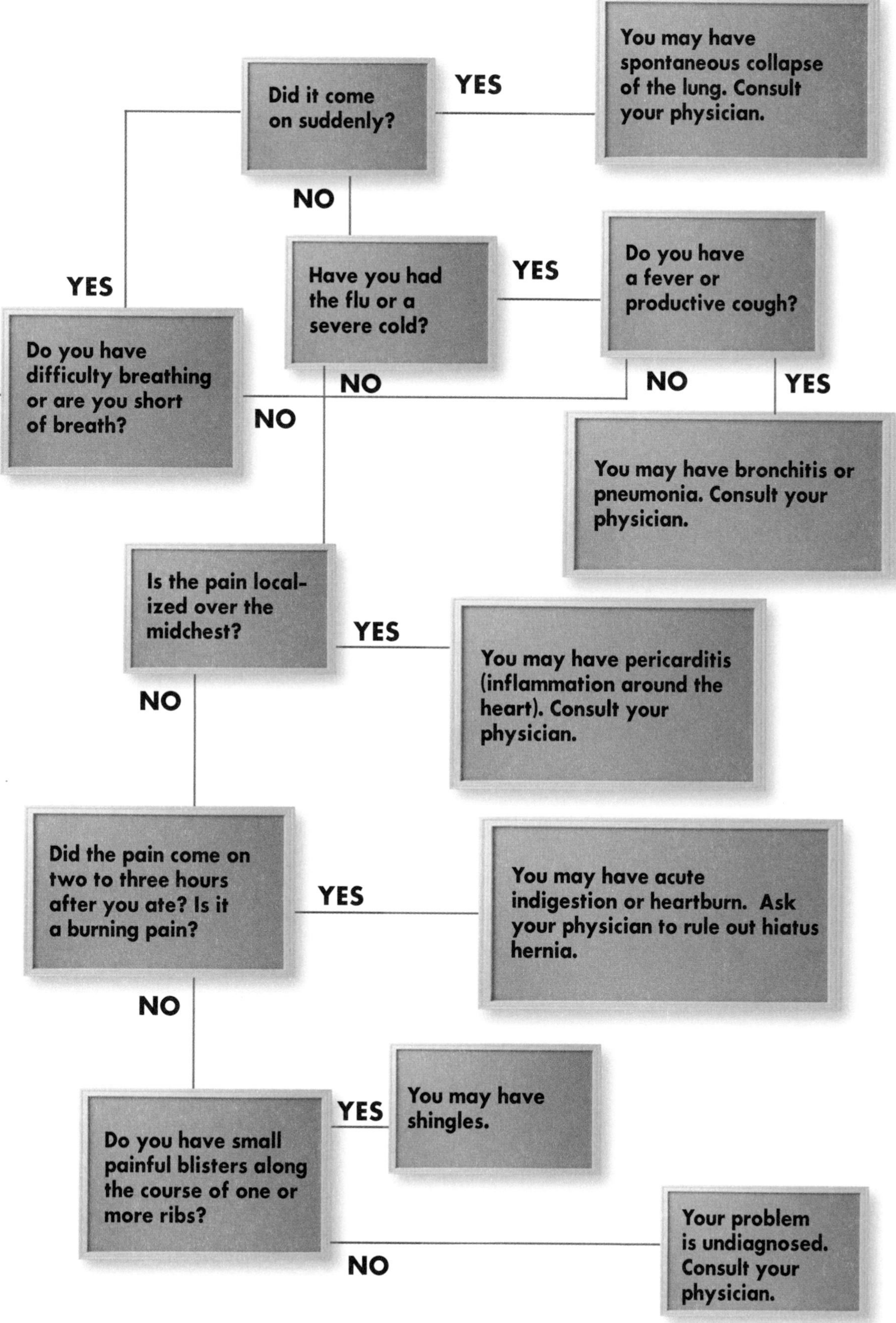
Did it come on suddenly?
YES
You may have spontaneous collapse of the lung. Consult your physician.
NO
Have you had the flu or a severe cold?
YES
Do you have a fever or productive cough?
YES
Do you have difficulty breathing or are you short of breath?
NO
NO
NO
YES
You may have bronchitis or pneumonia. Consult your physician.
Is the pain localized over the midchest?
YES
You may have pericarditis (inflammation around the heart). Consult your physician.
NO
Did the pain come on two to three hours after you ate? Is it a burning pain?
YES
You may have acute indigestion or heartburn. Ask your physician to rule out hiatus hernia.
NO
Do you have small painful blisters along the course of one or more ribs?
YES
You may have shingles.
NO
Your problem is undiagnosed. Consult your physician.

Cough

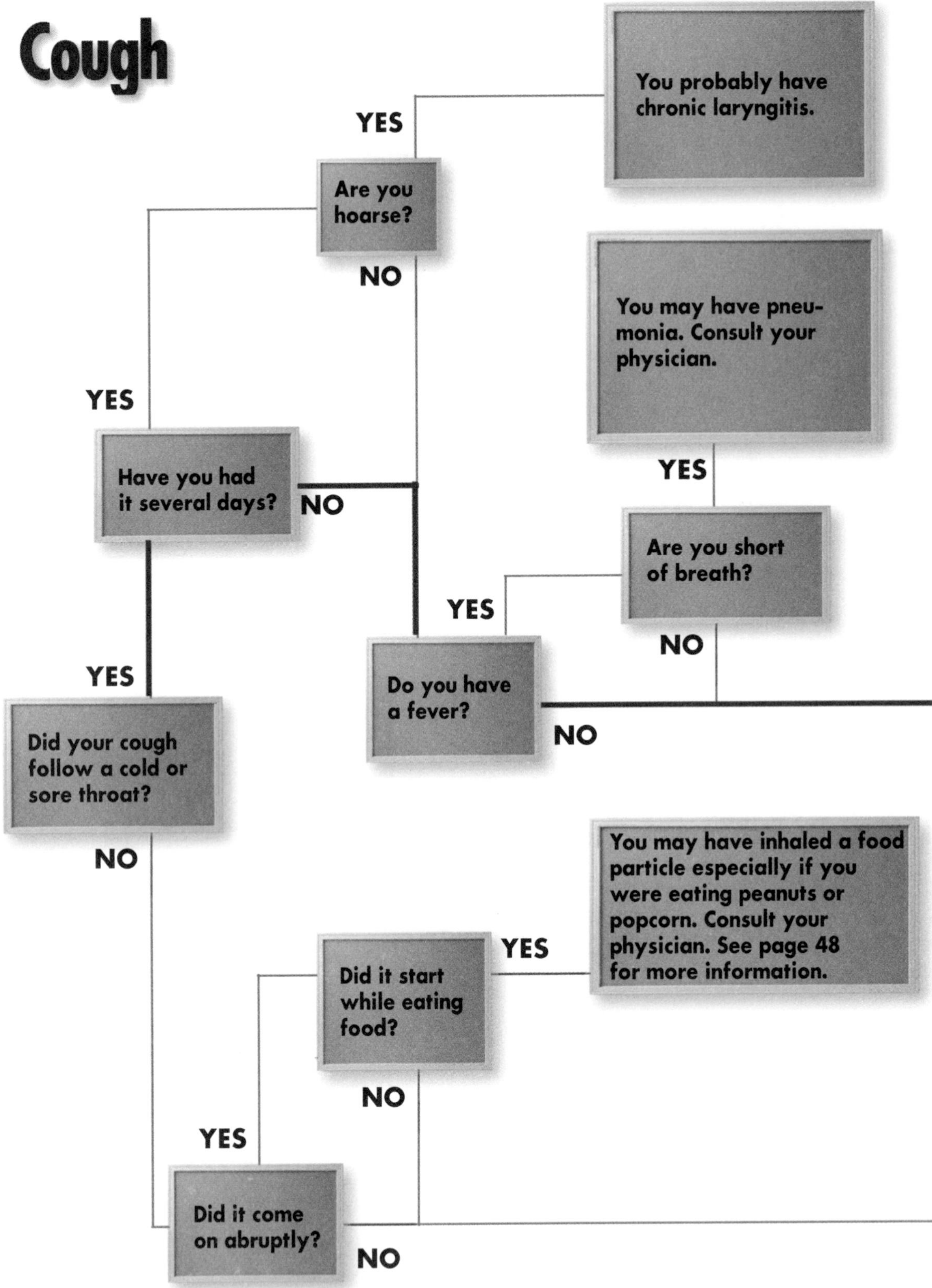

Are you hoarse?
YES
You probably have chronic laryngitis.
NO
YES
Have you had it several days?
NO
Do you have a fever?
YES
Are you short of breath?
YES
You may have pneumonia. Consult your physician.
NO
NO
YES
Did your cough follow a cold or sore throat?
NO
Did it come on abruptly?
YES
Did it start while eating food?
YES
You may have inhaled a food particle especially if you were eating peanuts or popcorn. Consult your physician. See page 48 for more information.
NO
NO

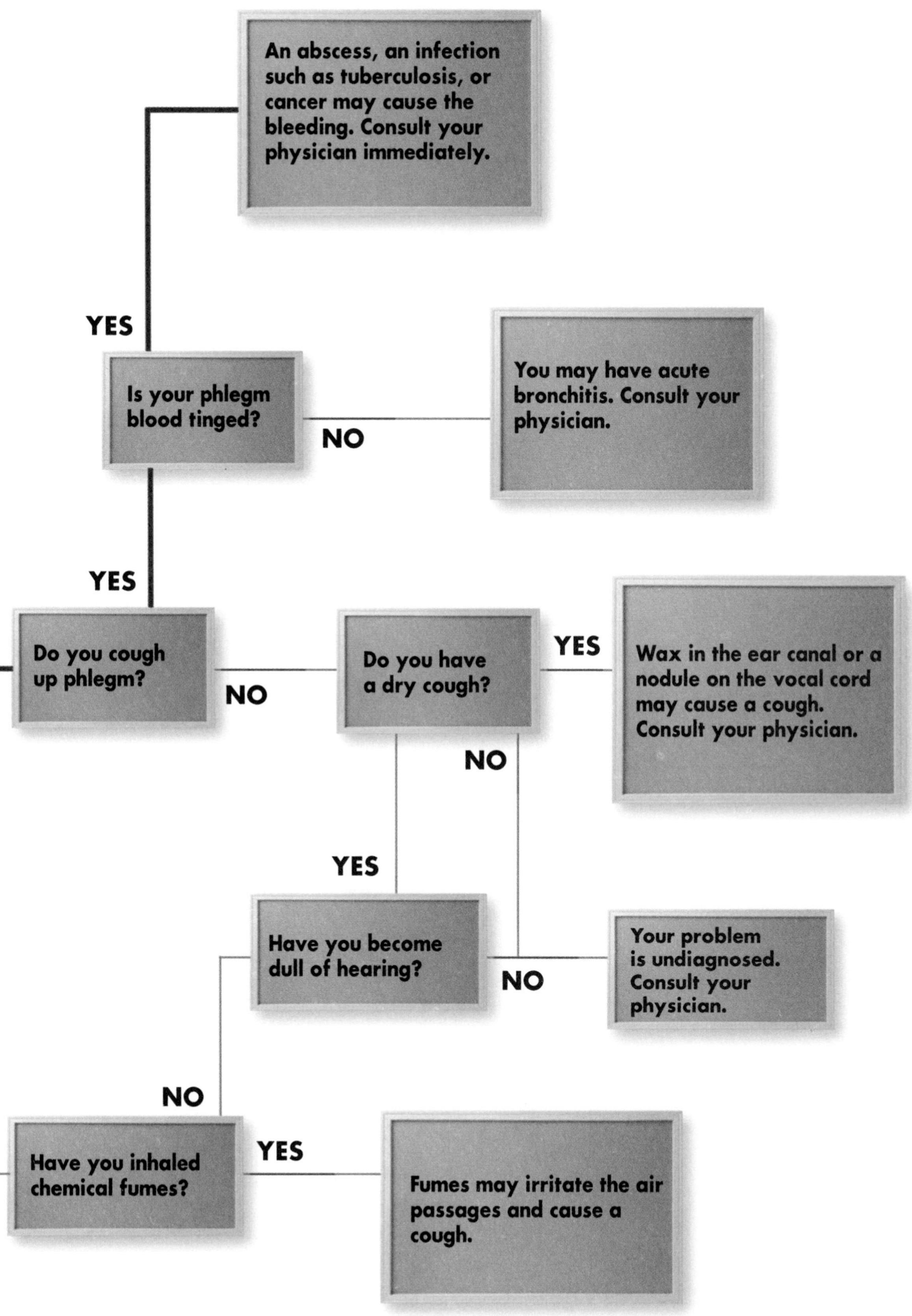
An abscess, an infection such as tuberculosis, or cancer may cause the bleeding. Consult your physician immediately.
YES
Is your phlegm blood tinged?
NO
You may have acute bronchitis. Consult your physician.
YES
Do you cough up phlegm?
NO
Do you have a dry cough?
YES
Wax in the ear canal or a nodule on the vocal cord may cause a cough. Consult your physician.
NO
YES
Have you become dull of hearing?
NO
Your problem is undiagnosed. Consult your physician.
NO
Have you inhaled chemical fumes?
YES
Fumes may irritate the air passages and cause a cough.

Earache

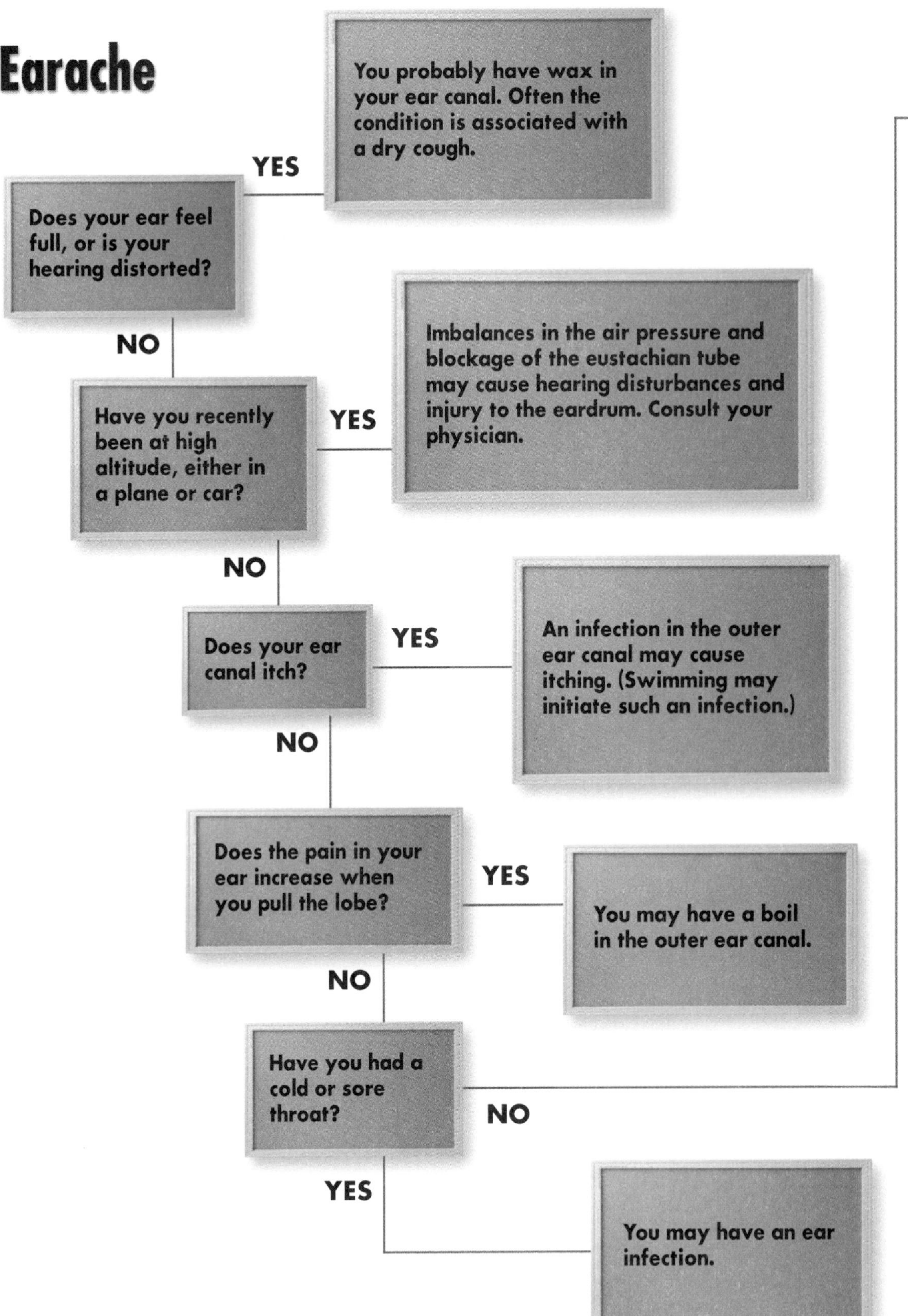
You probably have wax in your ear canal. Often the condition is associated with a dry cough.
YES
Does your ear feel full, or is your hearing distorted?
NO
Imbalances in the air pressure and blockage of the eustachian tube may cause hearing disturbances and injury to the eardrum. Consult your physician.
Have you recently been at high altitude, either in a plane or car?
YES
NO
Does your ear canal itch?
YES
An infection in the outer ear canal may cause itching. (Swimming may initiate such an infection.)
NO
Does the pain in your ear increase when you pull the lobe?
YES
You may have a boil in the outer ear canal.
NO
Have you had a cold or sore throat?
NO
YES
You may have an ear infection.

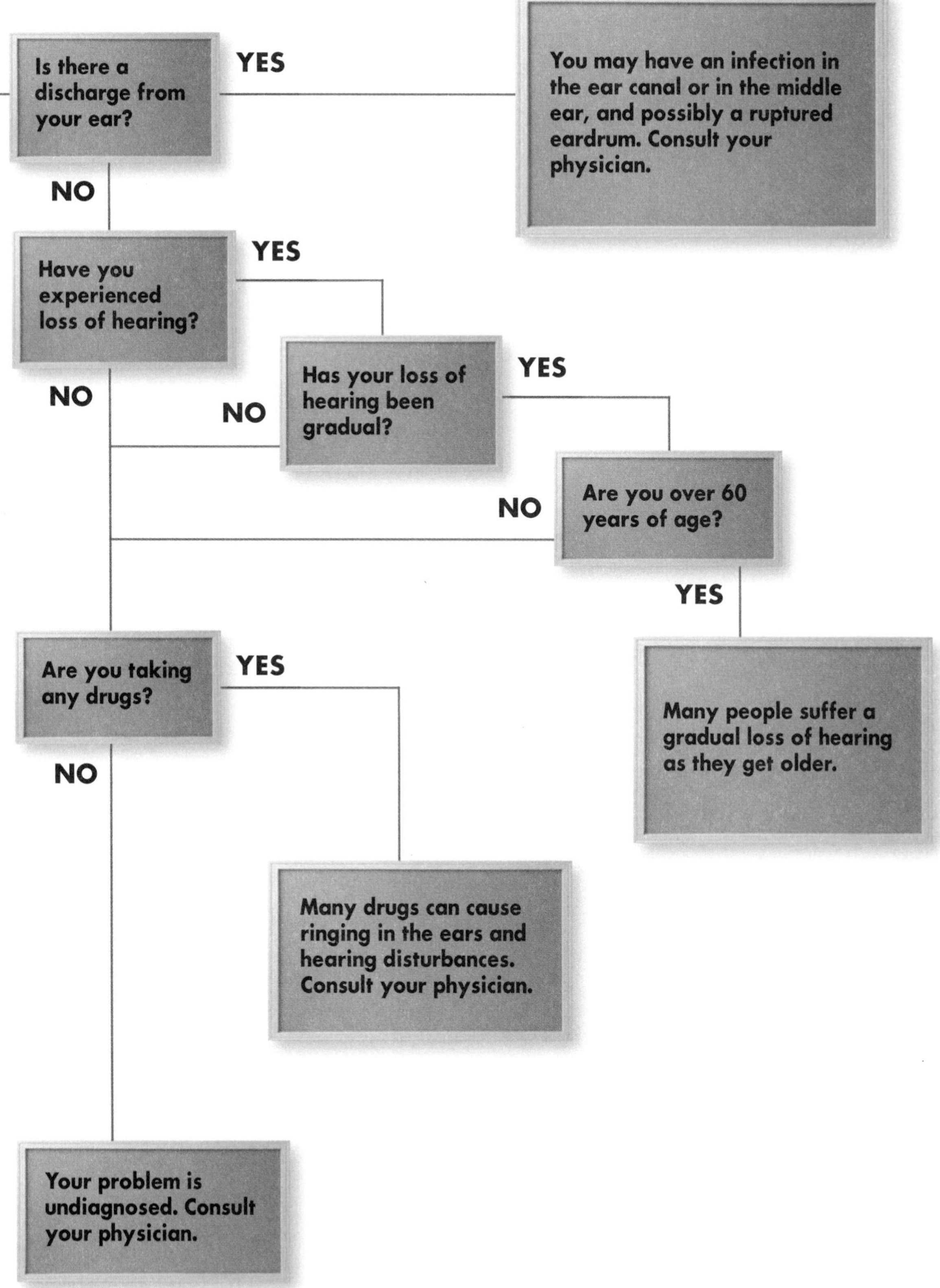
Is there a discharge from your ear?
YES
You may have an infection in the ear canal or in the middle ear, and possibly a ruptured eardrum. Consult your physician.
NO
Have you experienced loss of hearing?
YES
Has your loss of hearing been gradual?
NO
NO
YES
Are you over 60 years of age?
NO
YES
Many people suffer a gradual loss of hearing as they get older.
Are you taking any drugs?
YES
Many drugs can cause ringing in the ears and hearing disturbances. Consult your physician.
NO
Your problem is undiagnosed. Consult your physician.

Eye problems

You probably have conjuctivitis. Consult your physician.
YES
Is the white of your eye red?
YES
Is there a thick, sticky discharge?
NO
NO
YES
Did you injure your eye?
Does your eye hurt?
YES
NO
You may have injured your cornea. Consult your physician.
NO
Do your eyelids turn inward or outward?
NO
Are tears running from your eye?
YES
YES
Does it feel as if you have sand in your eye?
YES
You probably have a small object in your eye—sand, an eyelash, sawdust, etc. See pages 45-47 for what to do.
Entropion and ectropion are eyelid disorders. Consult your physician.

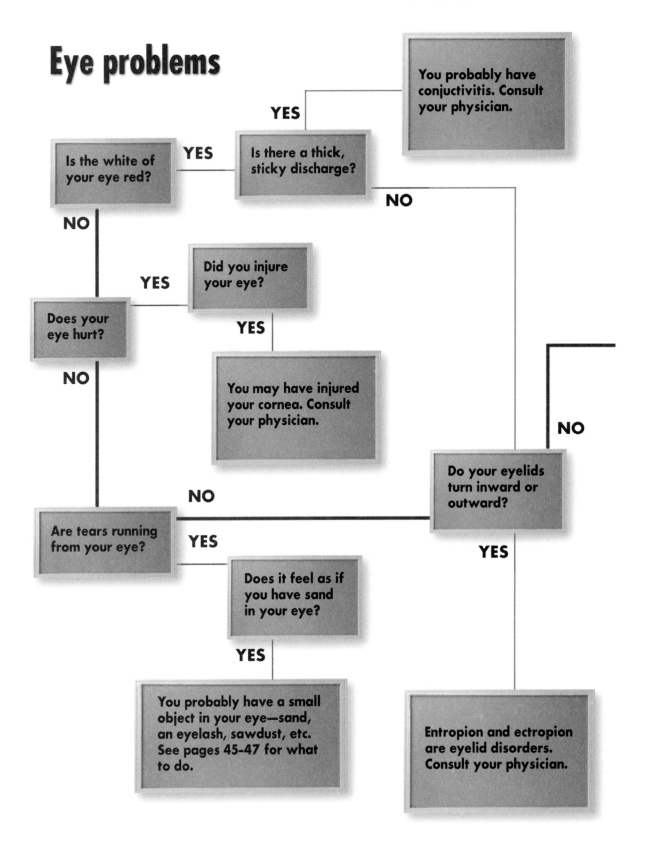

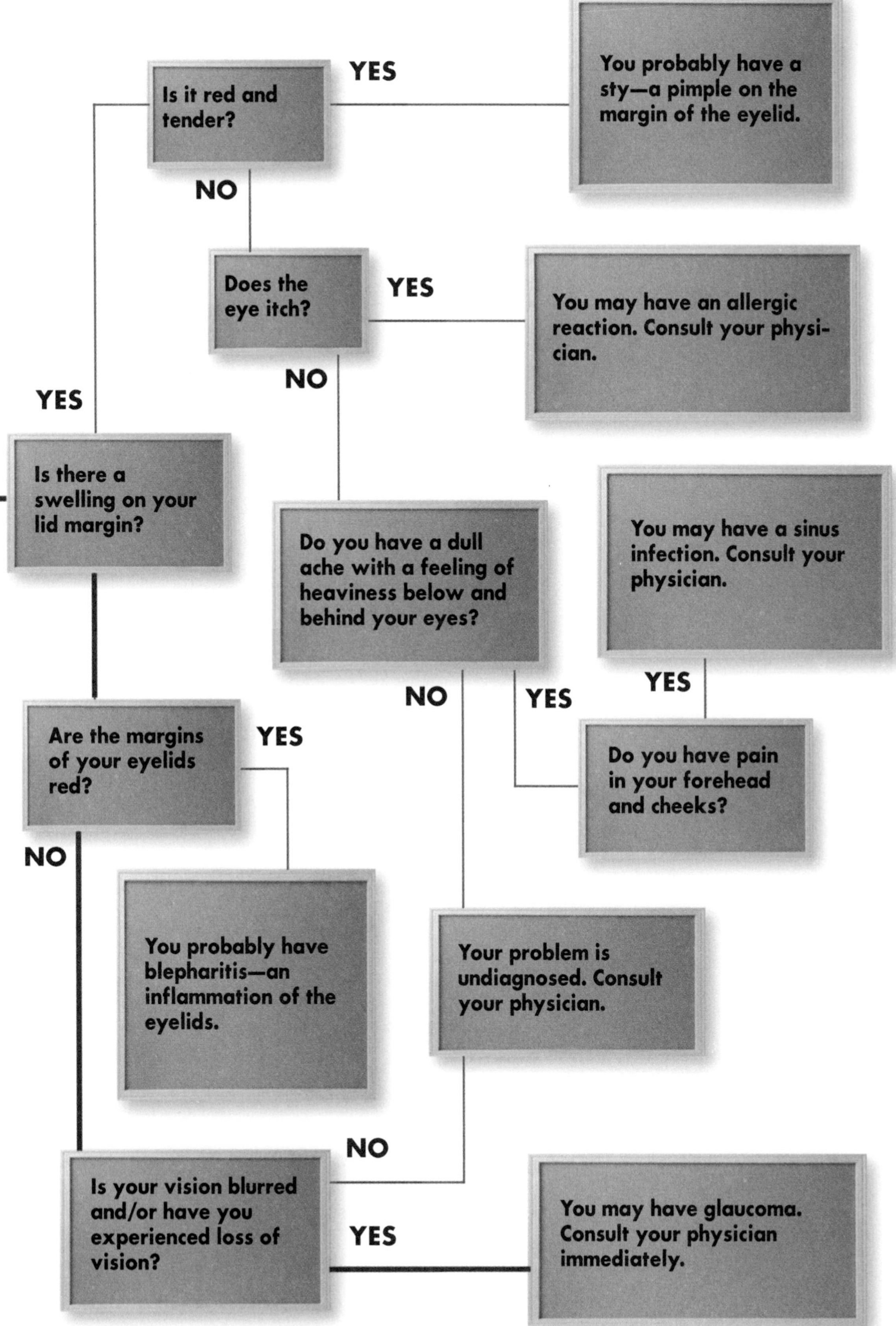
Is it red and tender?
YES
You probably have a sty—a pimple on the margin of the eyelid.
NO
Does the eye itch?
YES
You may have an allergic reaction. Consult your physician.
NO
YES
Is there a swelling on your lid margin?
Do you have a dull ache with a feeling of heaviness below and behind your eyes?
You may have a sinus infection. Consult your physician.
NO
YES
YES
Are the margins of your eyelids red?
YES
Do you have pain in your forehead and cheeks?
NO
You probably have blepharitis—an inflammation of the eyelids.
Your problem is undiagnosed. Consult your physician.
NO
Is your vision blurred and/or have you experienced loss of vision?
YES
You may have glaucoma. Consult your physician immediately.

Fever (adult)

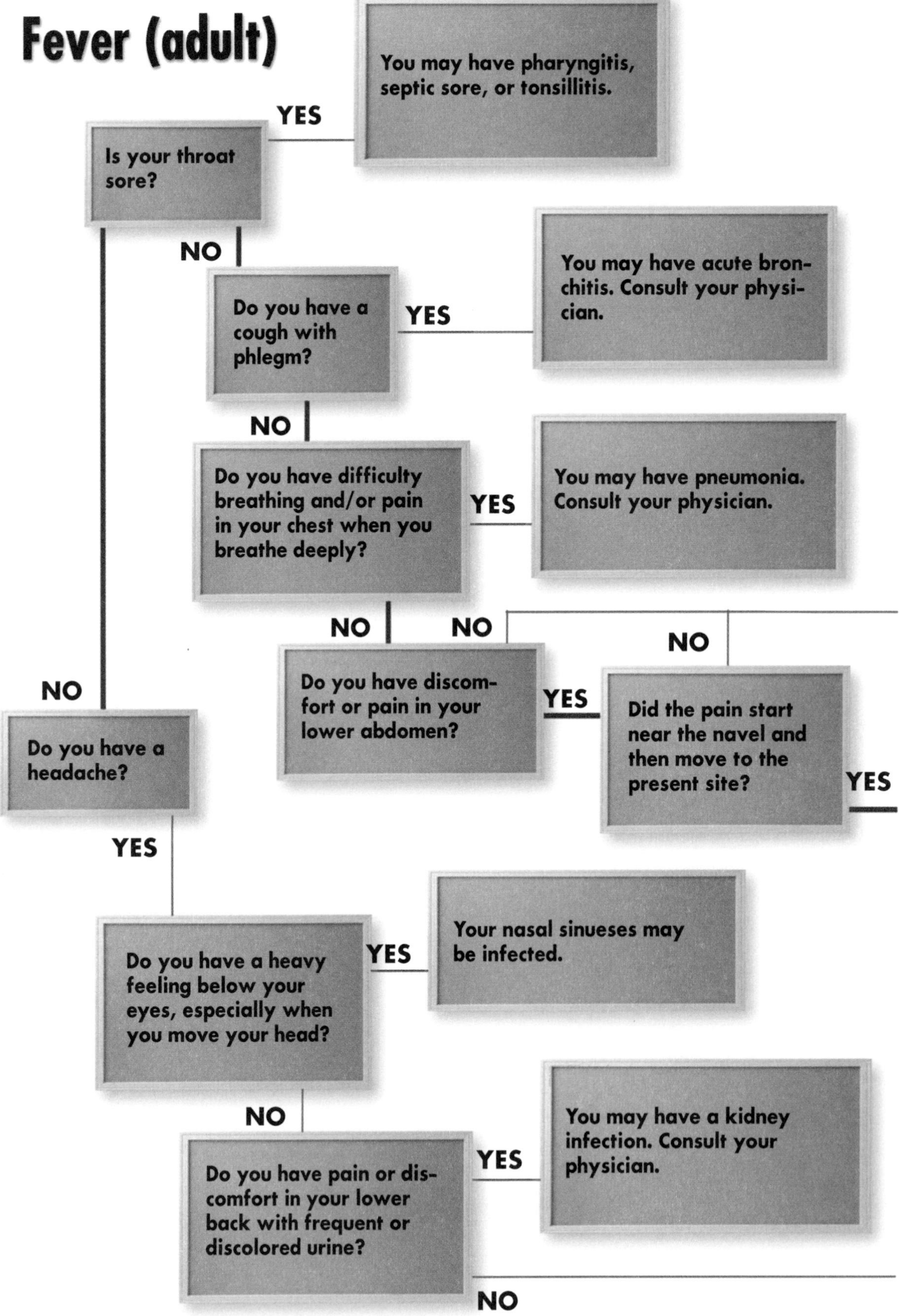

Is your throat sore?
YES
You may have pharyngitis, septic sore, or tonsillitis.
NO
Do you have a cough with phlegm?
YES
You may have acute bronchitis. Consult your physician.
NO
Do you have difficulty breathing and/or pain in your chest when you breathe deeply?
YES
You may have pneumonia. Consult your physician.
NO
NO
Do you have discomfort or pain in your lower abdomen?
YES
NO
Did the pain start near the navel and then move to the present site?
YES
NO
Do you have a headache?
YES
Do you have a heavy feeling below your eyes, especially when you move your head?
YES
Your nasal sinueses may be infected.
NO
Do you have pain or discomfort in your lower back with frequent or discolored urine?
YES
You may have a kidney infection. Consult your physician.
NO

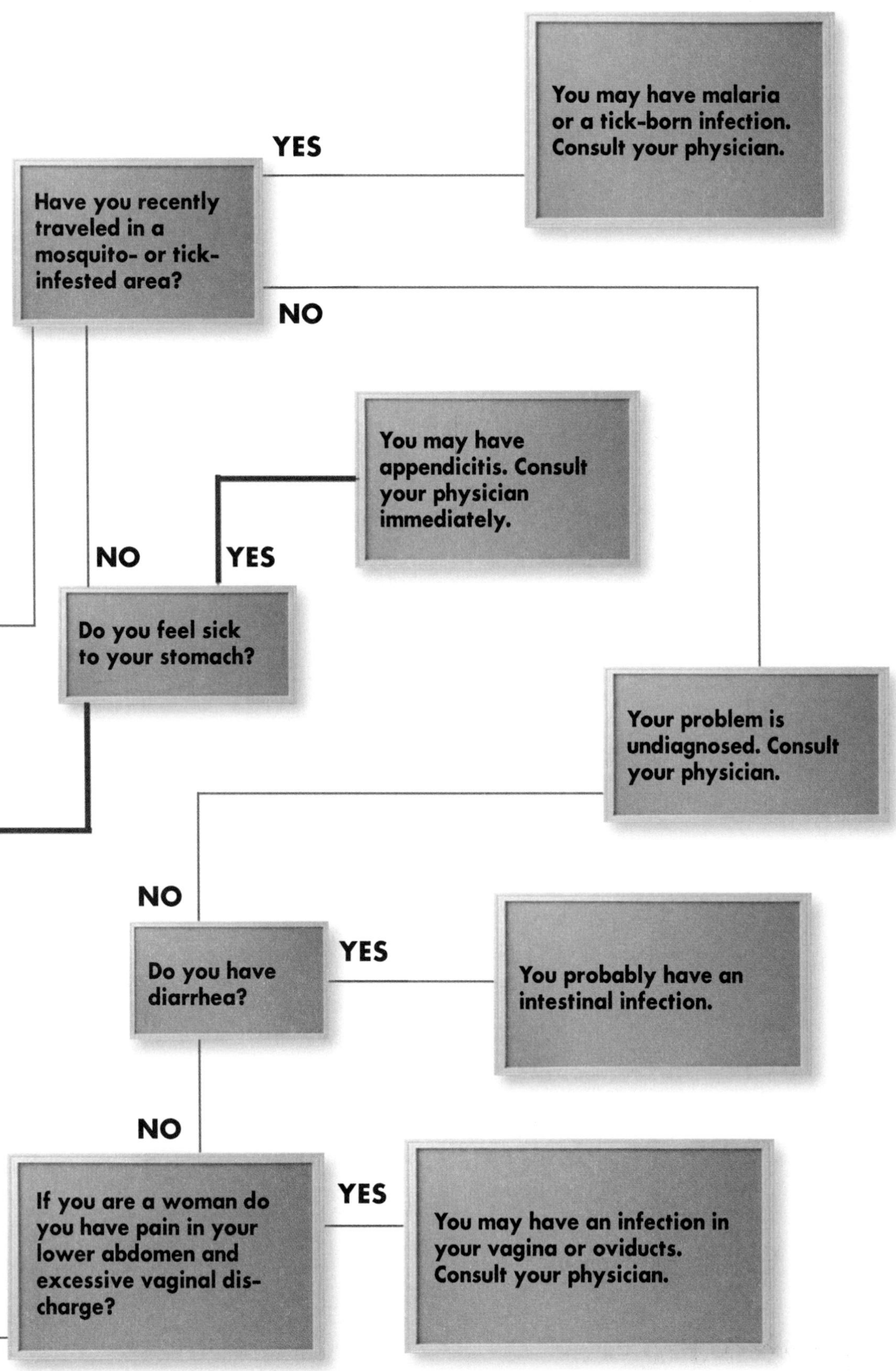

You may have malaria or a tick-born infection. Consult your physician.
YES
Have you recently traveled in a mosquito- or tick-infested area?
NO
You may have appendicitis. Consult your physician immediately.
NO
YES
Do you feel sick to your stomach?
Your problem is undiagnosed. Consult your physician.
NO
YES
Do you have diarrhea?
You probably have an intestinal infection.
NO
YES
If you are a woman do you have pain in your lower abdomen and excessive vaginal dis-charge?
You may have an infection in your vagina or oviducts. Consult your physician.

Fever (infant or child)

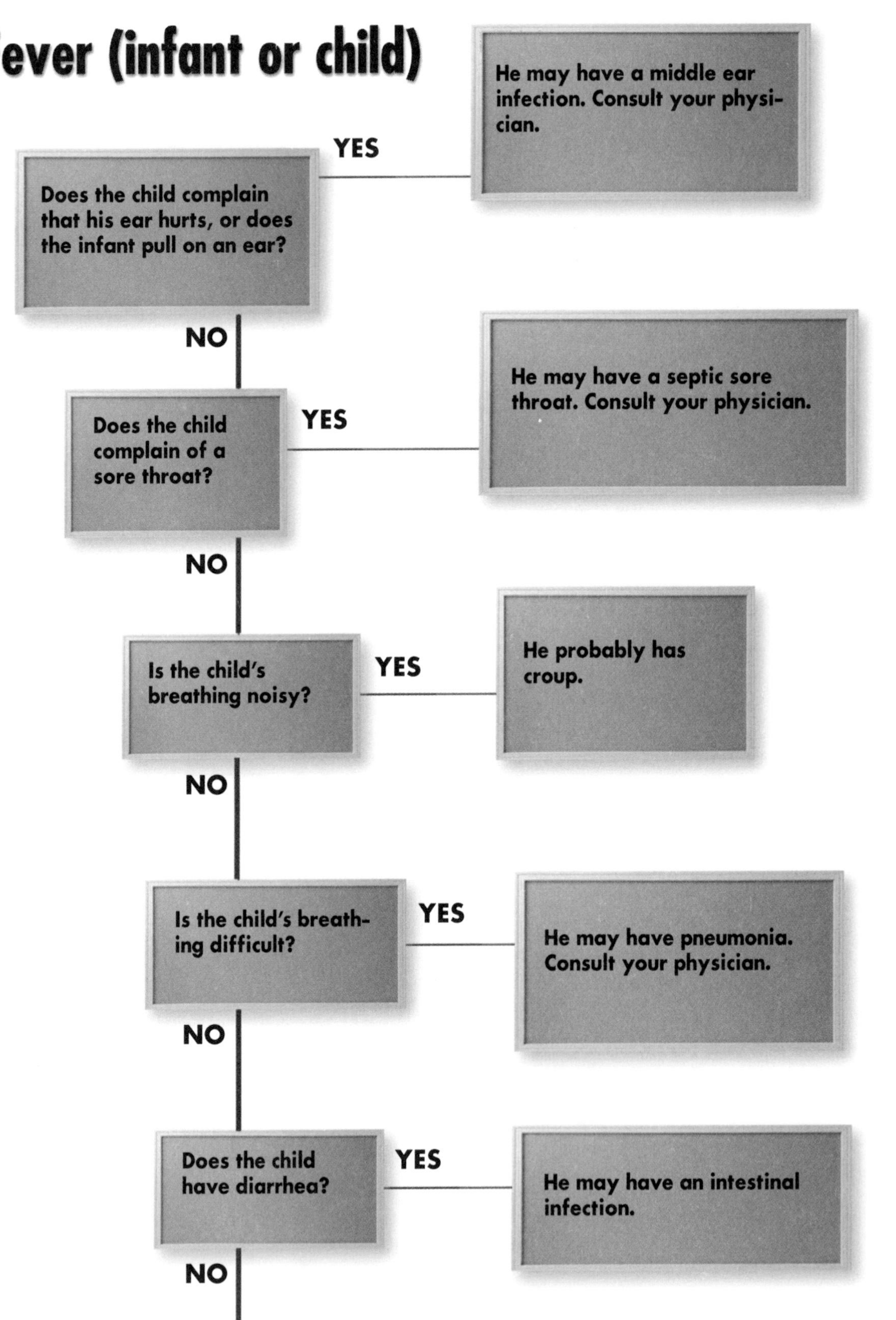

Does the child complain that his ear hurts, or does the infant pull on an ear?
YES
He may have a middle ear infection. Consult your physician.
NO
Does the child complain of a sore throat?
YES
He may have a septic sore throat. Consult your physician.
NO
Is the child's breathing noisy?
YES
He probably has croup.
NO
Is the child's breathing difficult?
YES
He may have pneumonia. Consult your physician.
NO
Does the child have diarrhea?
YES
He may have an intestinal infection.
NO

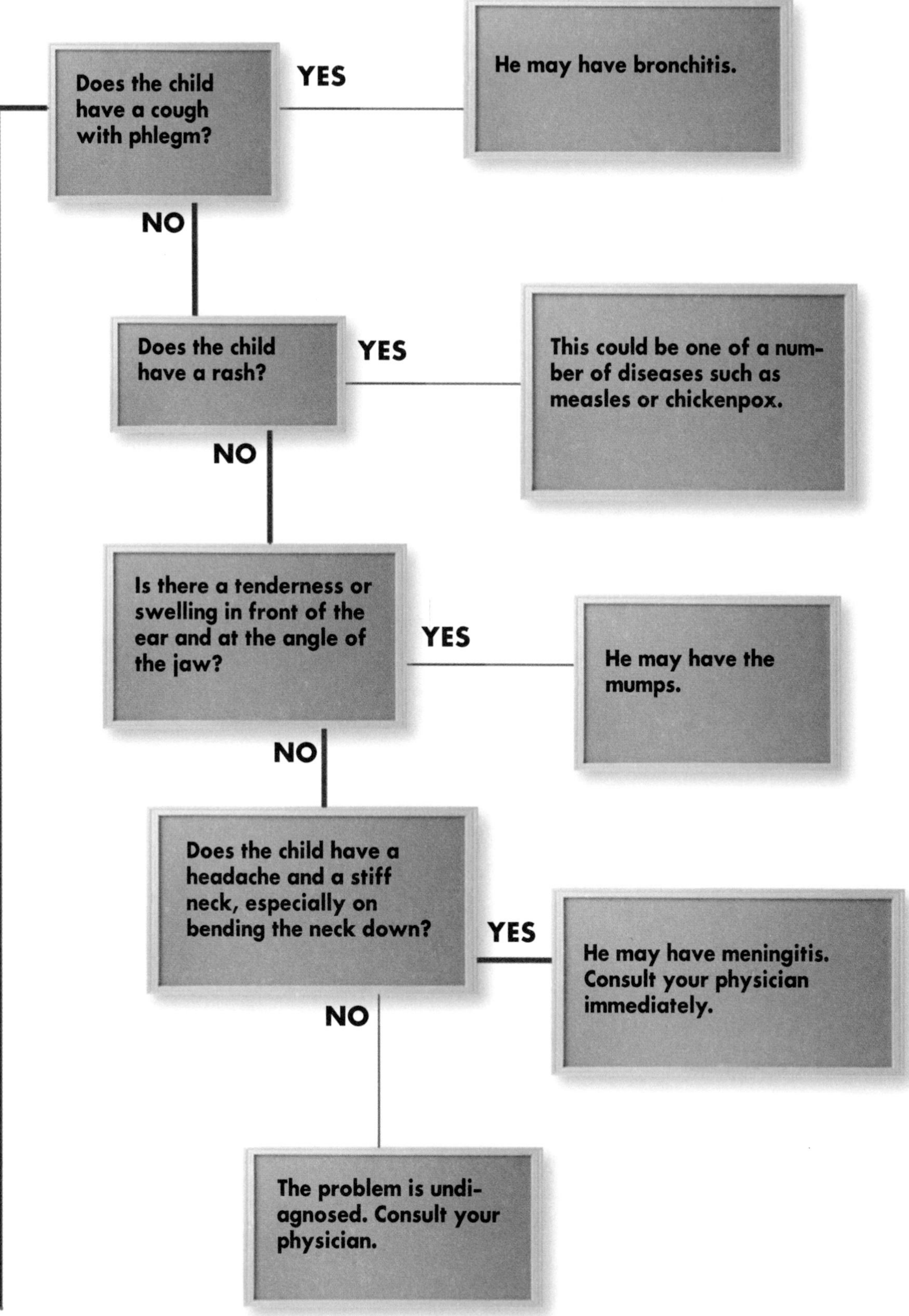
Does the child have a cough with phlegm?
YES
He may have bronchitis.
NO
Does the child have a rash?
YES
This could be one of a number of diseases such as measles or chickenpox.
NO
Is there a tenderness or swelling in front of the ear and at the angle of the jaw?
YES
He may have the mumps.
NO
Does the child have a headache and a stiff neck, especially on bending the neck down?
YES
He may have meningitis. Consult your physician immediately.
NO
The problem is undiagnosed. Consult your physician.

Headache

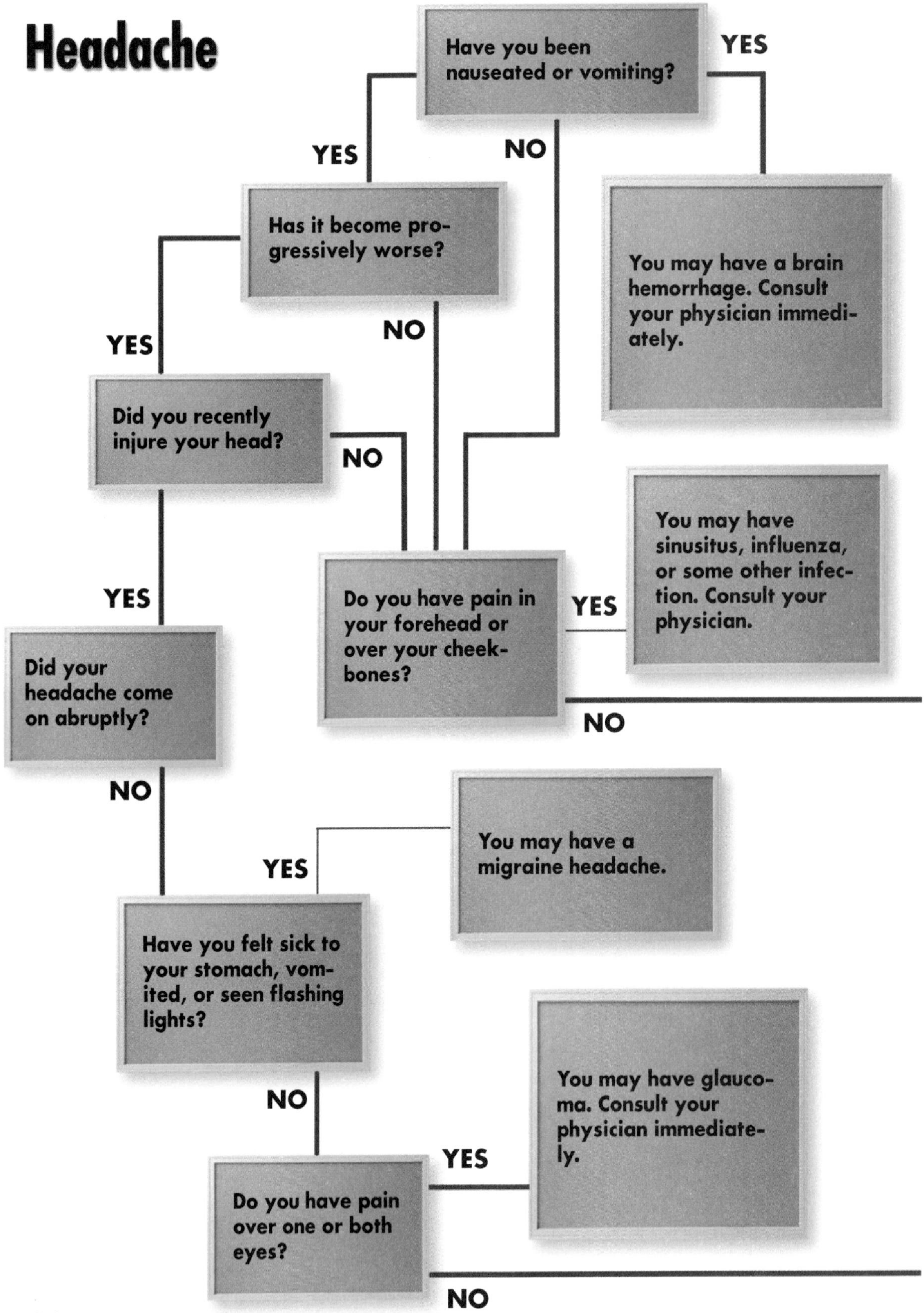

Have you been nauseated or vomiting?
YES
You may have a brain hemorrhage. Consult your physician immediately.
YES
NO
Has it become progressively worse?
YES
NO
Did you recently injure your head?
NO
YES
Did your headache come on abruptly?
Do you have pain in your forehead or over your cheekbones?
YES
You may have sinusitus, influenza, or some other infection. Consult your physician.
NO
NO
YES
You may have a migraine headache.
Have you felt sick to your stomach, vomited, or seen flashing lights?
NO
YES
You may have glaucoma. Consult your physician immediately.
Do you have pain over one or both eyes?
NO

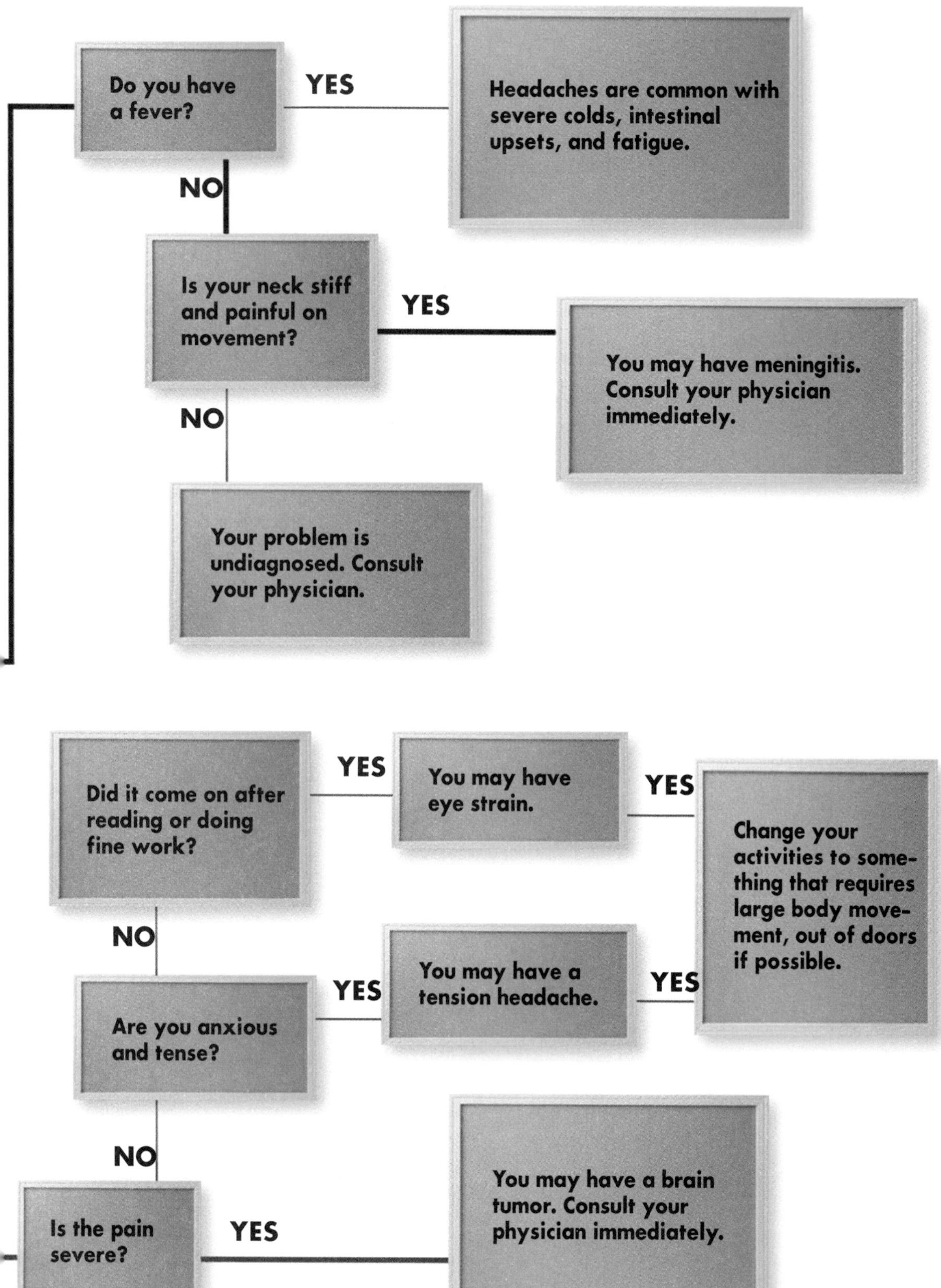
Do you have a fever?
YES
Headaches are common with severe colds, intestinal upsets, and fatigue.
NO
Is your neck stiff and painful on movement?
YES
You may have meningitis. Consult your physician immediately.
NO
Your problem is undiagnosed. Consult your physician.
Did it come on after reading or doing fine work?
YES
You may have eye strain.
YES
Change your activities to something that requires large body movement, out of doors if possible.
NO
Are you anxious and tense?
YES
You may have a tension headache.
YES
NO
Is the pain severe?
YES
You may have a brain tumor. Consult your physician immediately.

Itching

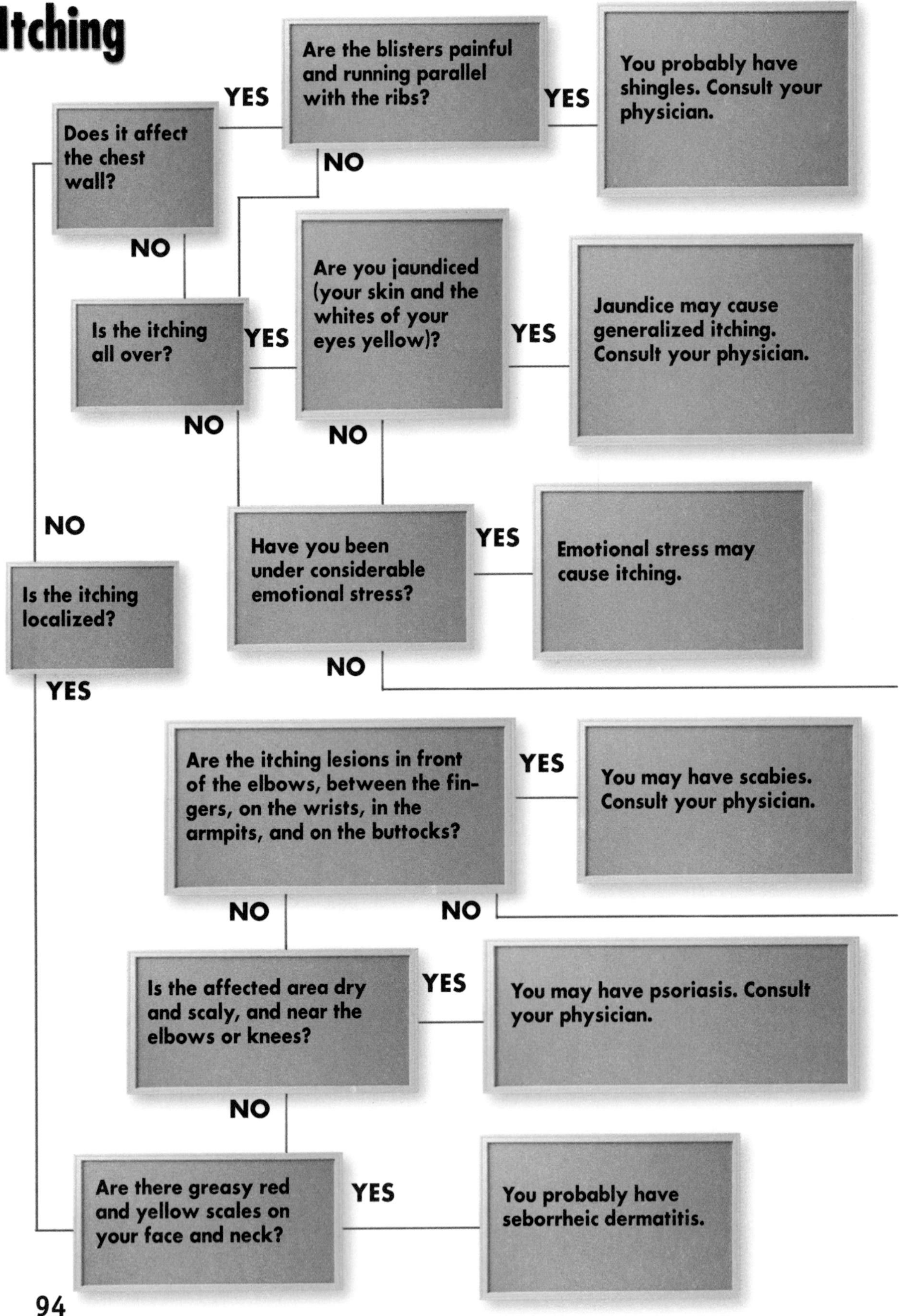

Does it affect the chest wall?
YES
Are the blisters painful and running parallel with the ribs?
YES
You probably have shingles. Consult your physician.
NO
NO
Is the itching all over?
YES
Are you jaundiced (your skin and the whites of your eyes yellow)?
YES
Jaundice may cause generalized itching. Consult your physician.
NO
NO
NO
Is the itching localized?
Have you been under considerable emotional stress?
YES
Emotional stress may cause itching.
NO
YES
Are the itching lesions in front of the elbows, between the fingers, on the wrists, in the armpits, and on the buttocks?
YES
You may have scabies. Consult your physician.
NO
NO
Is the affected area dry and scaly, and near the elbows or knees?
YES
You may have psoriasis. Consult your physician.
NO
Are there greasy red and yellow scales on your face and neck?
YES
You probably have seborrheic dermatitis.

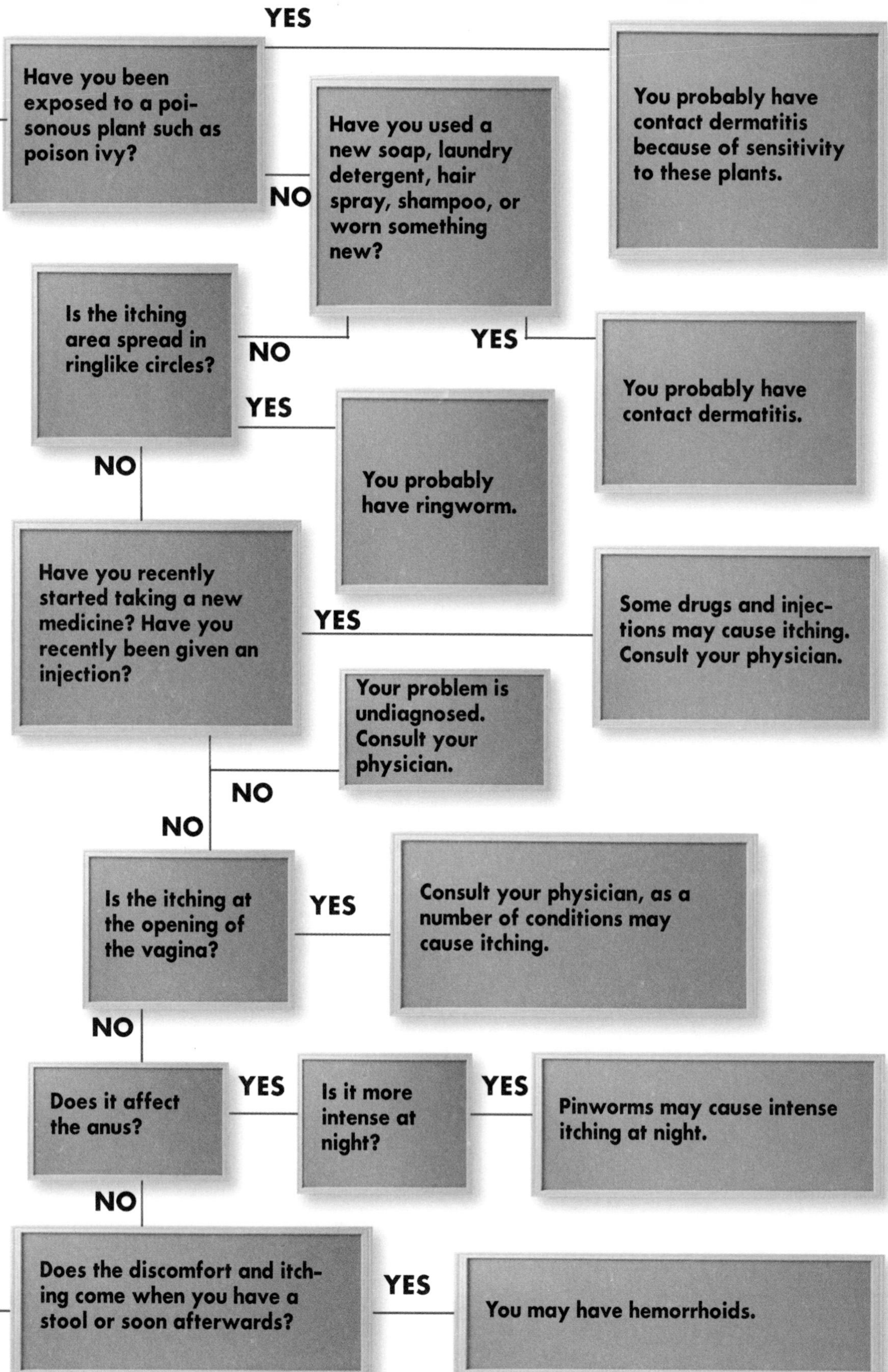
Have you been exposed to a poisonous plant such as poison ivy?
YES
You probably have contact dermatitis because of sensitivity to these plants.
NO
Have you used a new soap, laundry detergent, hair spray, shampoo, or worn something new?
YES
You probably have contact dermatitis.
NO
Is the itching area spread in ringlike circles?
YES
You probably have ringworm.
NO
Have you recently started taking a new medicine? Have you recently been given an injection?
YES
Some drugs and injections may cause itching. Consult your physician.
NO
Your problem is undiagnosed. Consult your physician.
NO
Is the itching at the opening of the vagina?
YES
Consult your physician, as a number of conditions may cause itching.
NO
Does it affect the anus?
YES
Is it more intense at night?
YES
Pinworms may cause intense itching at night.
NO
Does the discomfort and itching come when you have a stool or soon afterwards?
YES
You may have hemorrhoids.

Joint pain

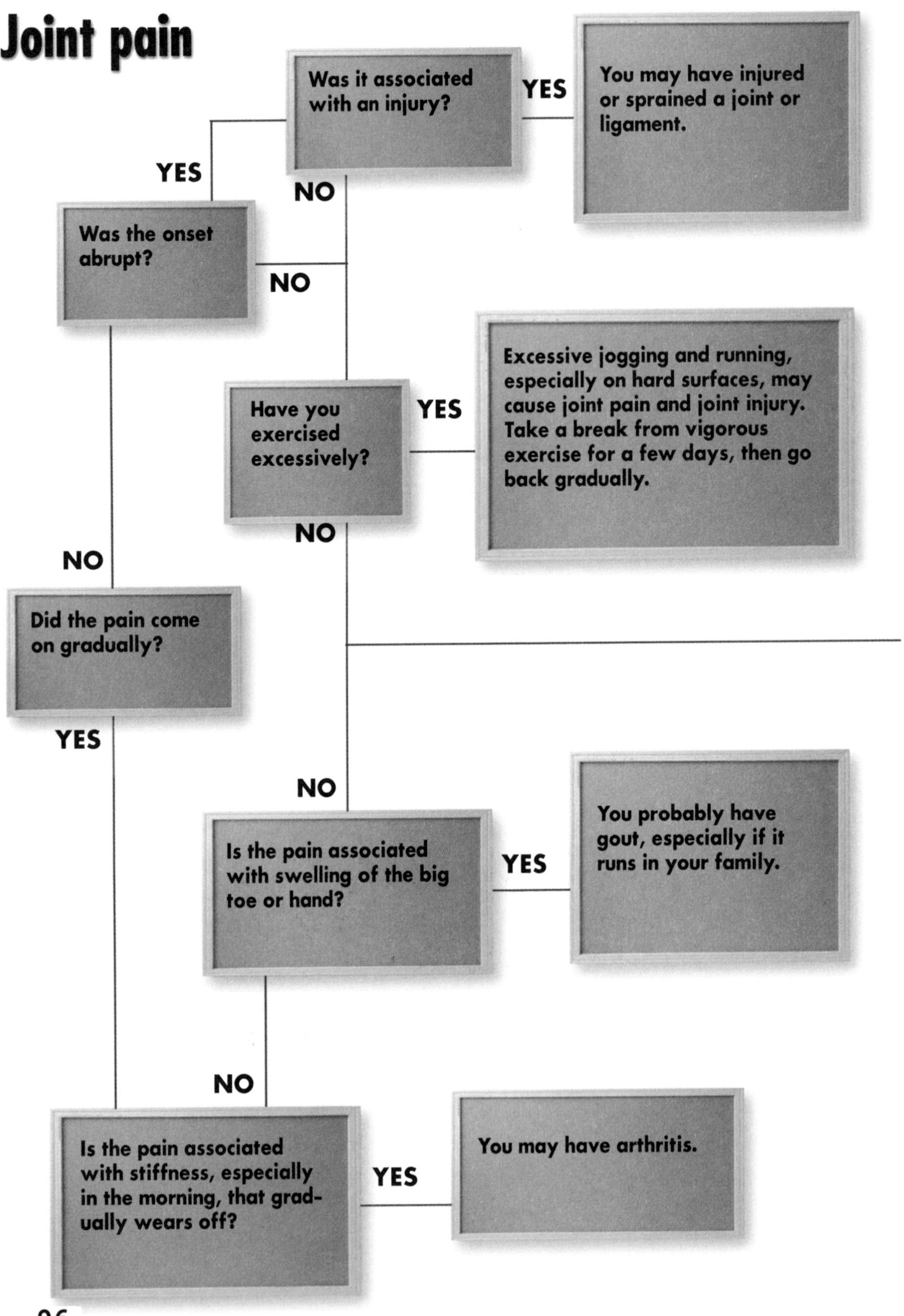
Was it associated with an injury?
YES
You may have injured or sprained a joint or ligament.
YES
NO
Was the onset abrupt?
NO
Have you exercised excessively?
YES
Excessive jogging and running, especially on hard surfaces, may cause joint pain and joint injury. Take a break from vigorous exercise for a few days, then go back gradually.
NO
NO
Did the pain come on gradually?
YES
NO
Is the pain associated with swelling of the big toe or hand?
YES
You probably have gout, especially if it runs in your family.
NO
Is the pain associated with stiffness, especially in the morning, that gradually wears off?
YES
You may have arthritis.

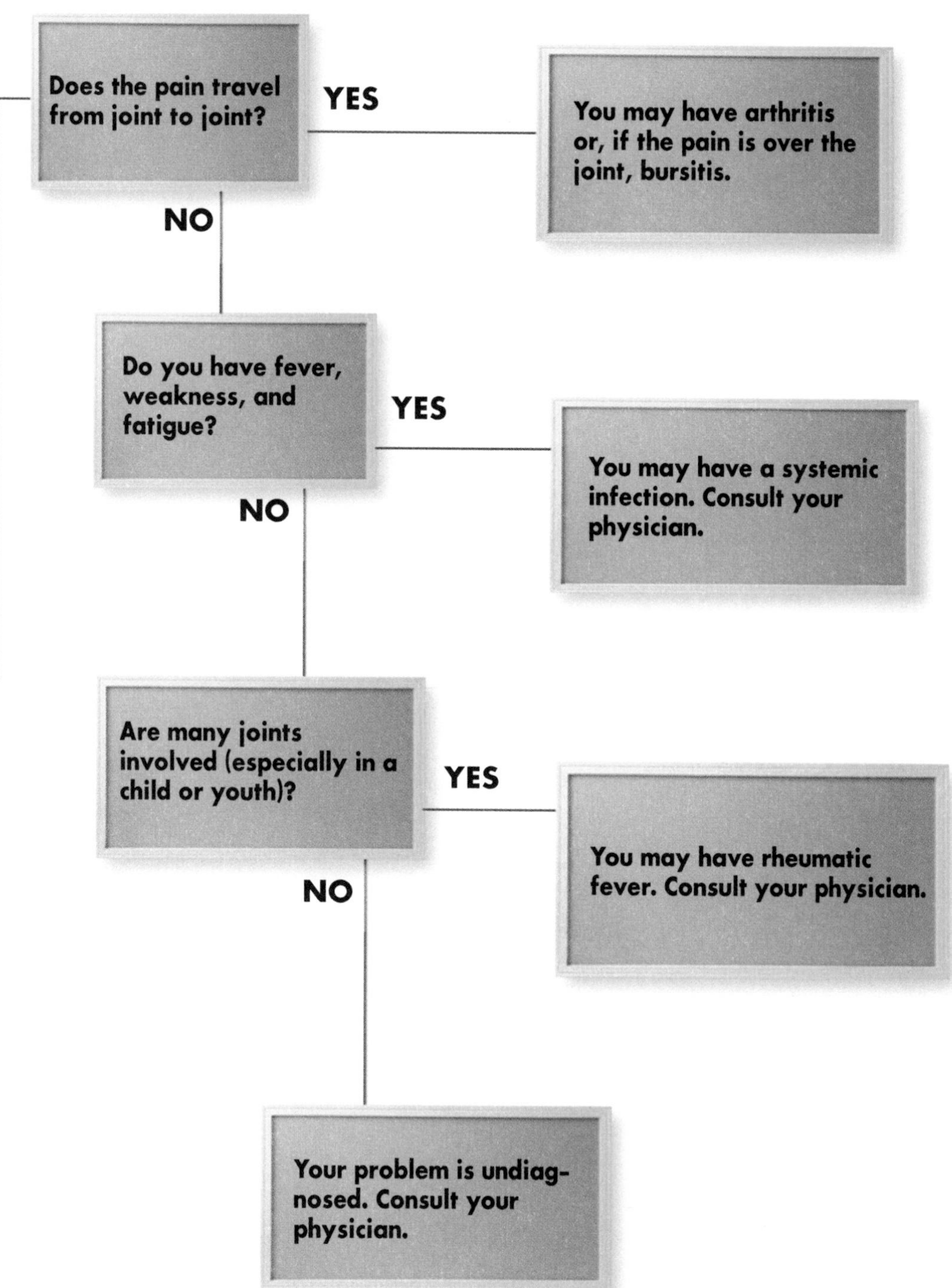
Does the pain travel from joint to joint?
YES
You may have arthritis or, if the pain is over the joint, bursitis.
NO
Do you have fever, weakness, and fatigue?
YES
You may have a systemic infection. Consult your physician.
NO
Are many joints involved (especially in a child or youth)?
YES
You may have rheumatic fever. Consult your physician.
NO
Your problem is undiagnosed. Consult your physician.

Neck pain

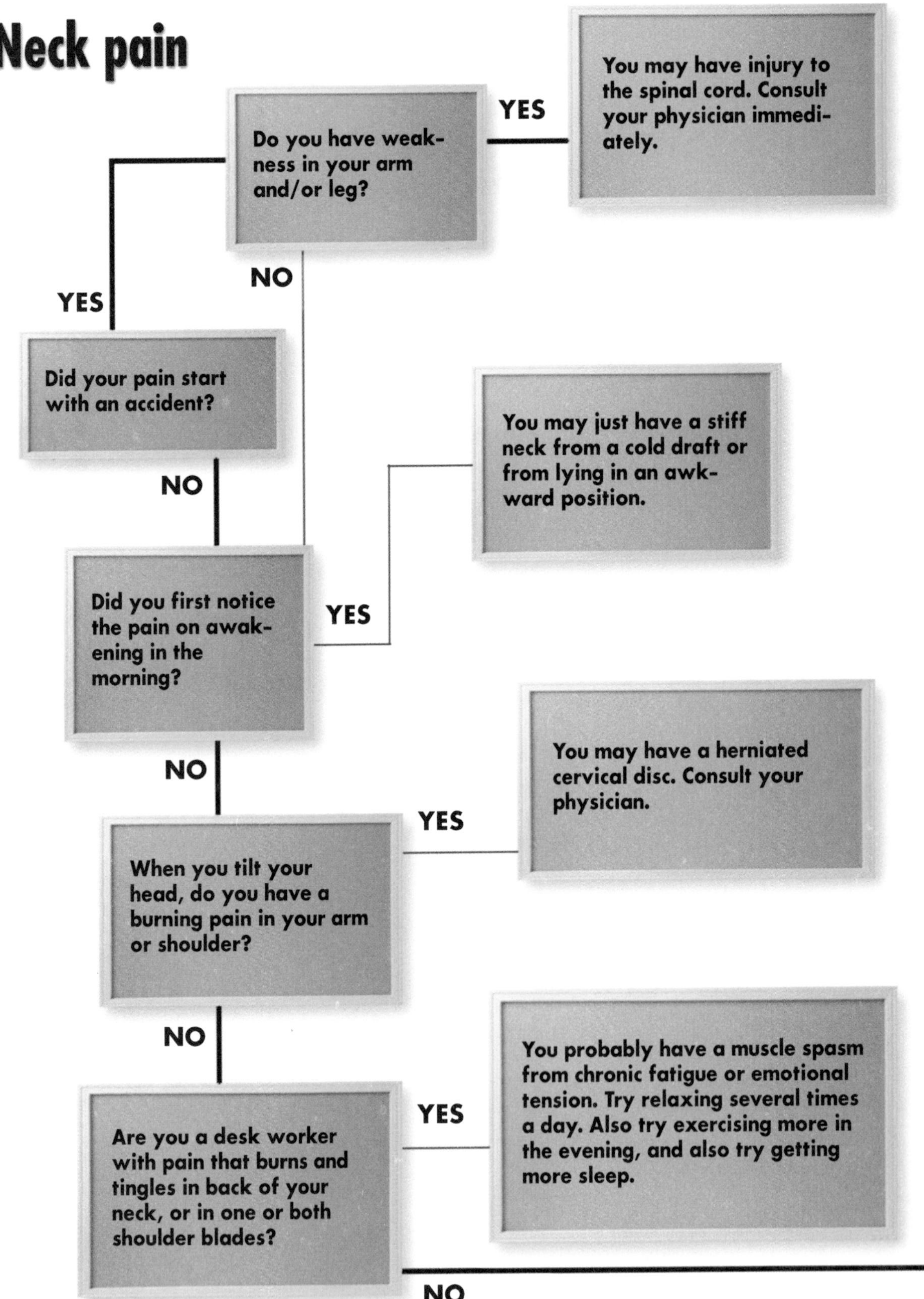

Do you have weakness in your arm and/or leg?
YES
You may have injury to the spinal cord. Consult your physician immediately.
NO
YES
Did your pain start with an accident?
NO
Did you first notice the pain on awakening in the morning?
YES
You may just have a stiff neck from a cold draft or from lying in an awkward position.
NO
When you tilt your head, do you have a burning pain in your arm or shoulder?
YES
You may have a herniated cervical disc. Consult your physician.
NO
Are you a desk worker with pain that burns and tingles in back of your neck, or in one or both shoulder blades?
YES
You probably have a muscle spasm from chronic fatigue or emotional tension. Try relaxing several times a day. Also try exercising more in the evening, and also try getting more sleep.
NO

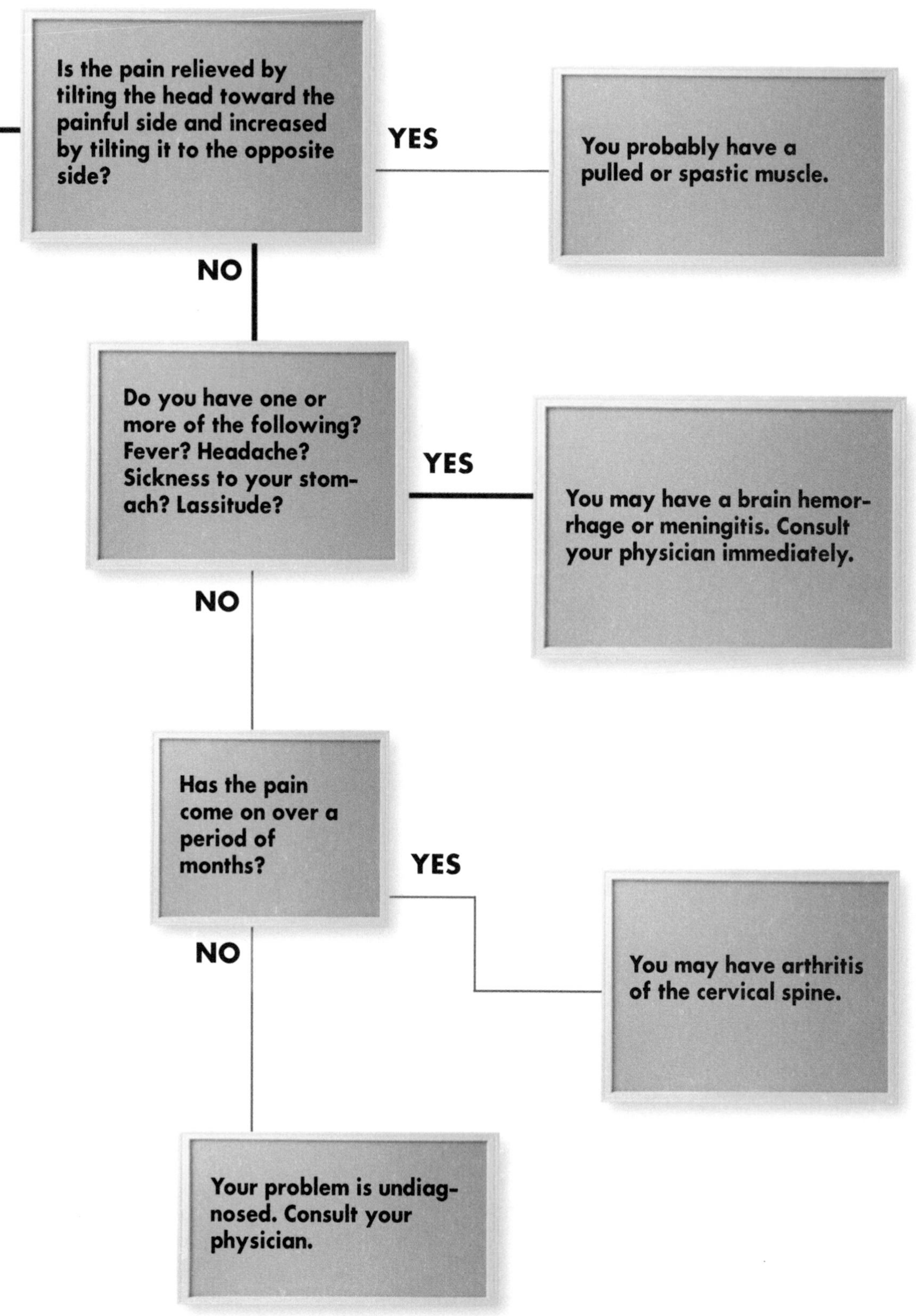

Is the pain relieved by tilting the head toward the painful side and increased by tilting it to the opposite side?
YES
You probably have a pulled or spastic muscle.
NO
Do you have one or more of the following? Fever? Headache? Sickness to your stomach? Lassitude?
YES
You may have a brain hemorrhage or meningitis. Consult your physician immediately.
NO
Has the pain come on over a period of months?
YES
You may have arthritis of the cervical spine.
NO
Your problem is undiagnosed. Consult your physician.

Sick feeling (malaise)

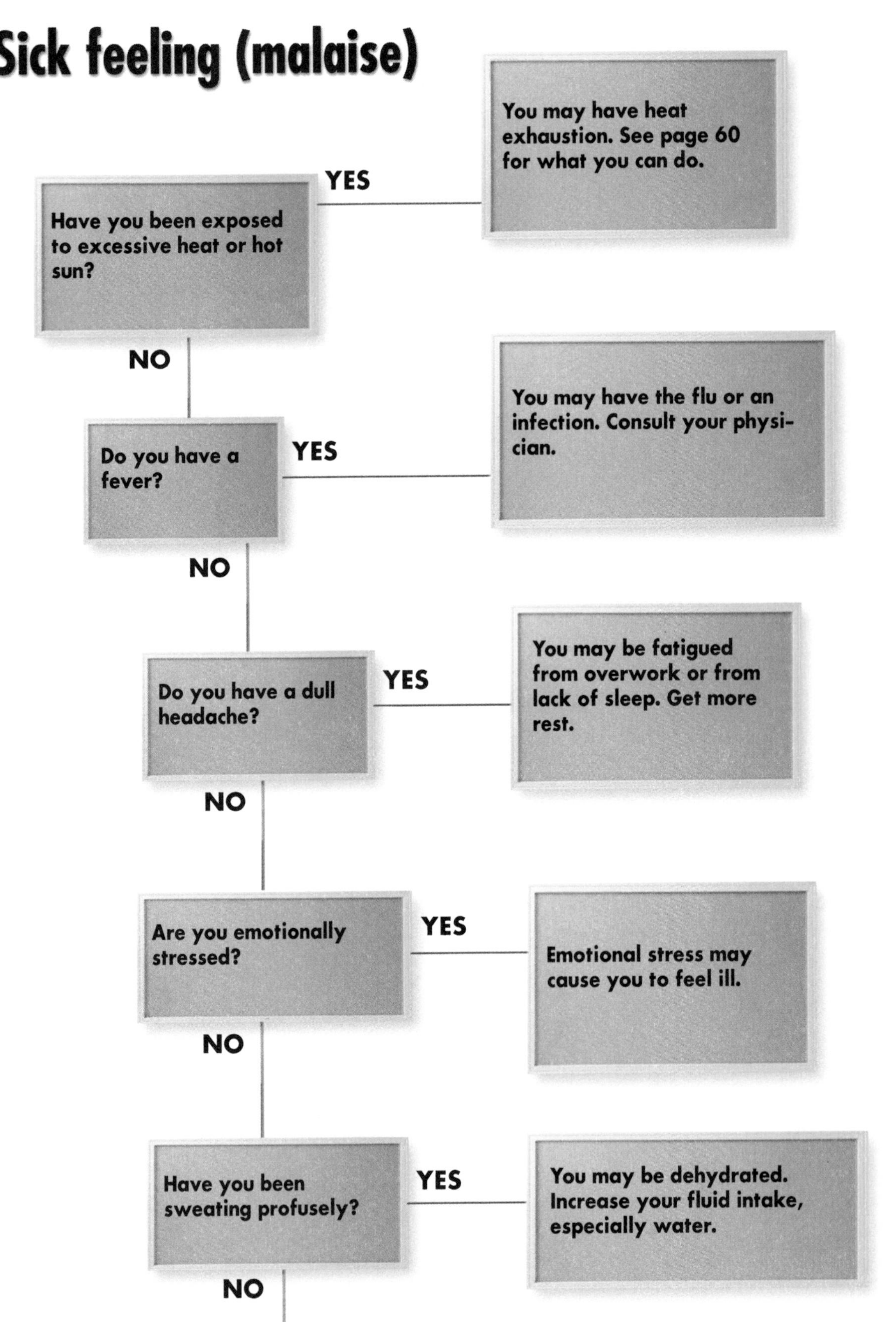

Have you been exposed to excessive heat or hot sun?
YES
You may have heat exhaustion. See page 60 for what you can do.
NO
Do you have a fever?
YES
You may have the flu or an infection. Consult your physician.
NO
Do you have a dull headache?
YES
You may be fatigued from overwork or from lack of sleep. Get more rest.
NO
Are you emotionally stressed?
YES
Emotional stress may cause you to feel ill.
NO
Have you been sweating profusely?
YES
You may be dehydrated. Increase your fluid intake, especially water.
NO

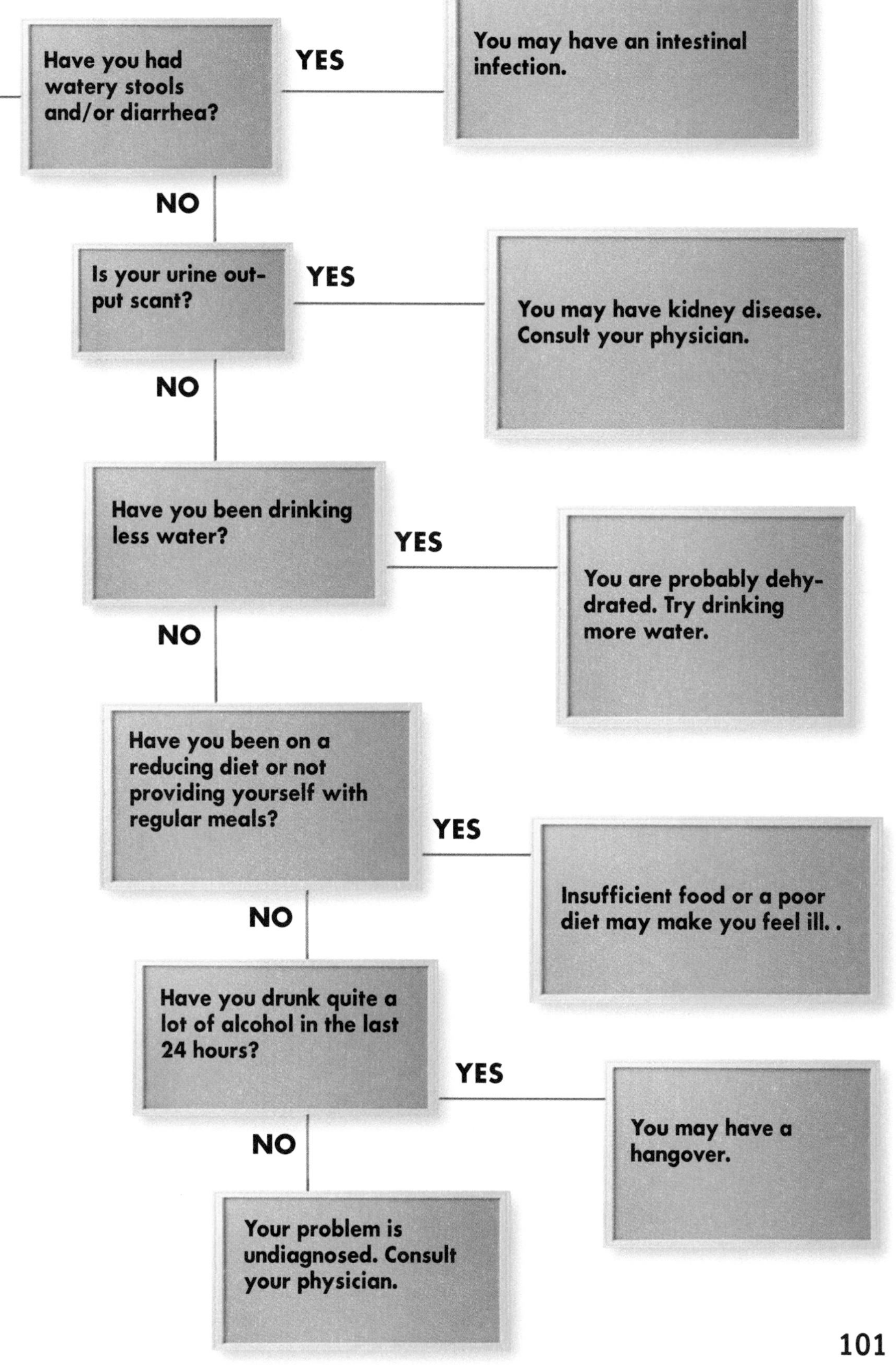
Have you had watery stools and/or diarrhea?
YES
You may have an intestinal infection.
NO
Is your urine output scant?
YES
You may have kidney disease. Consult your physician.
NO
Have you been drinking less water?
YES
You are probably dehydrated. Try drinking more water.
NO
Have you been on a reducing diet or not providing yourself with regular meals?
YES
Insufficient food or a poor diet may make you feel ill. .
NO
Have you drunk quite a lot of alcohol in the last 24 hours?
YES
You may have a hangover.
NO
Your problem is undiagnosed. Consult your physician.

Throat, sore

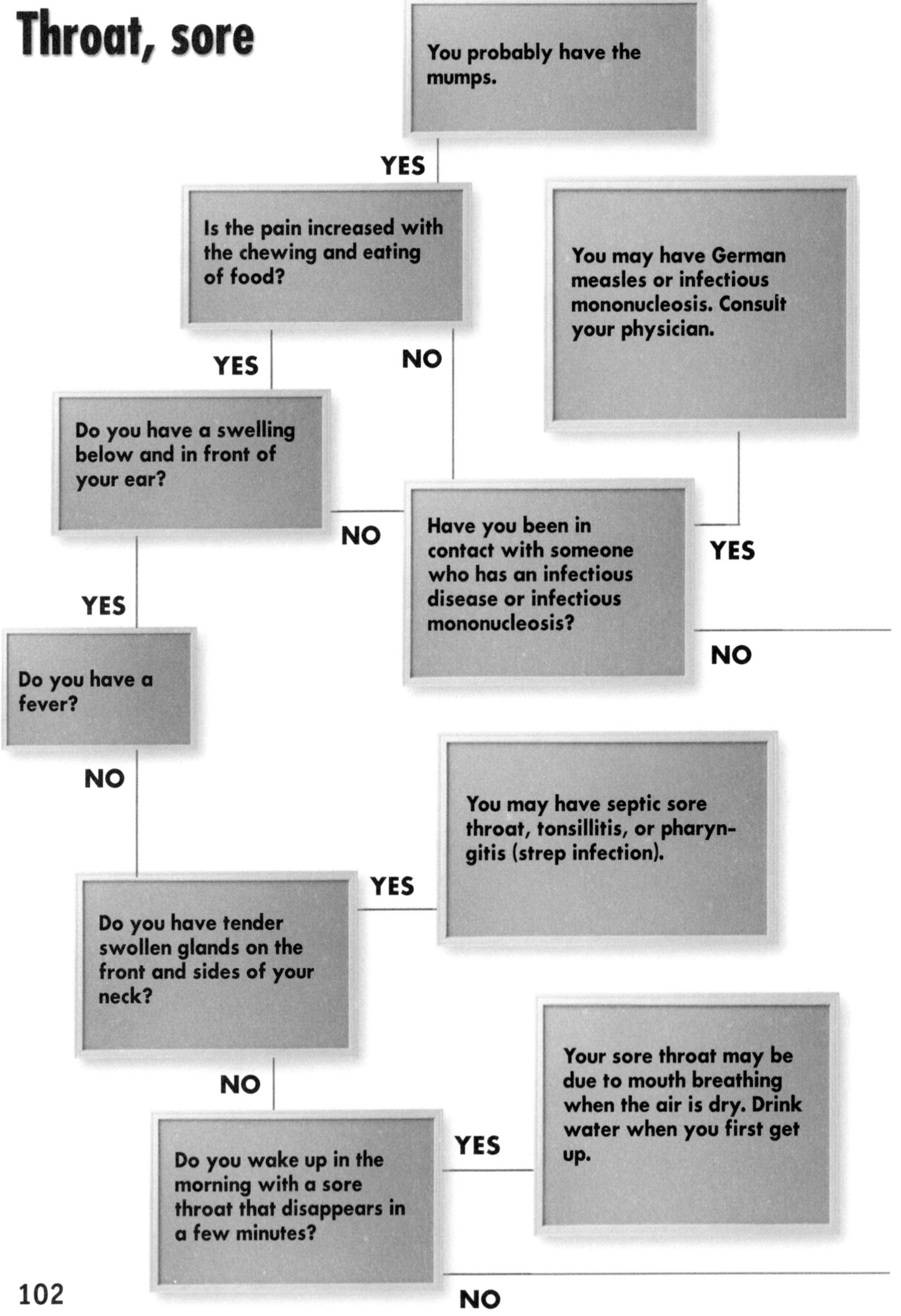

You probably have the mumps.
YES
Is the pain increased with the chewing and eating of food?
You may have German measles or infectious mononucleosis. Consult your physician.
YES
NO
Do you have a swelling below and in front of your ear?
NO
Have you been in contact with someone who has an infectious disease or infectious mononucleosis?
YES
NO
YES
Do you have a fever?
NO
You may have septic sore throat, tonsillitis, or pharyngitis (strep infection).
YES
Do you have tender swollen glands on the front and sides of your neck?
Your sore throat may be due to mouth breathing when the air is dry. Drink water when you first get up.
NO
Do you wake up in the morning with a sore throat that disappears in a few minutes?
YES
NO

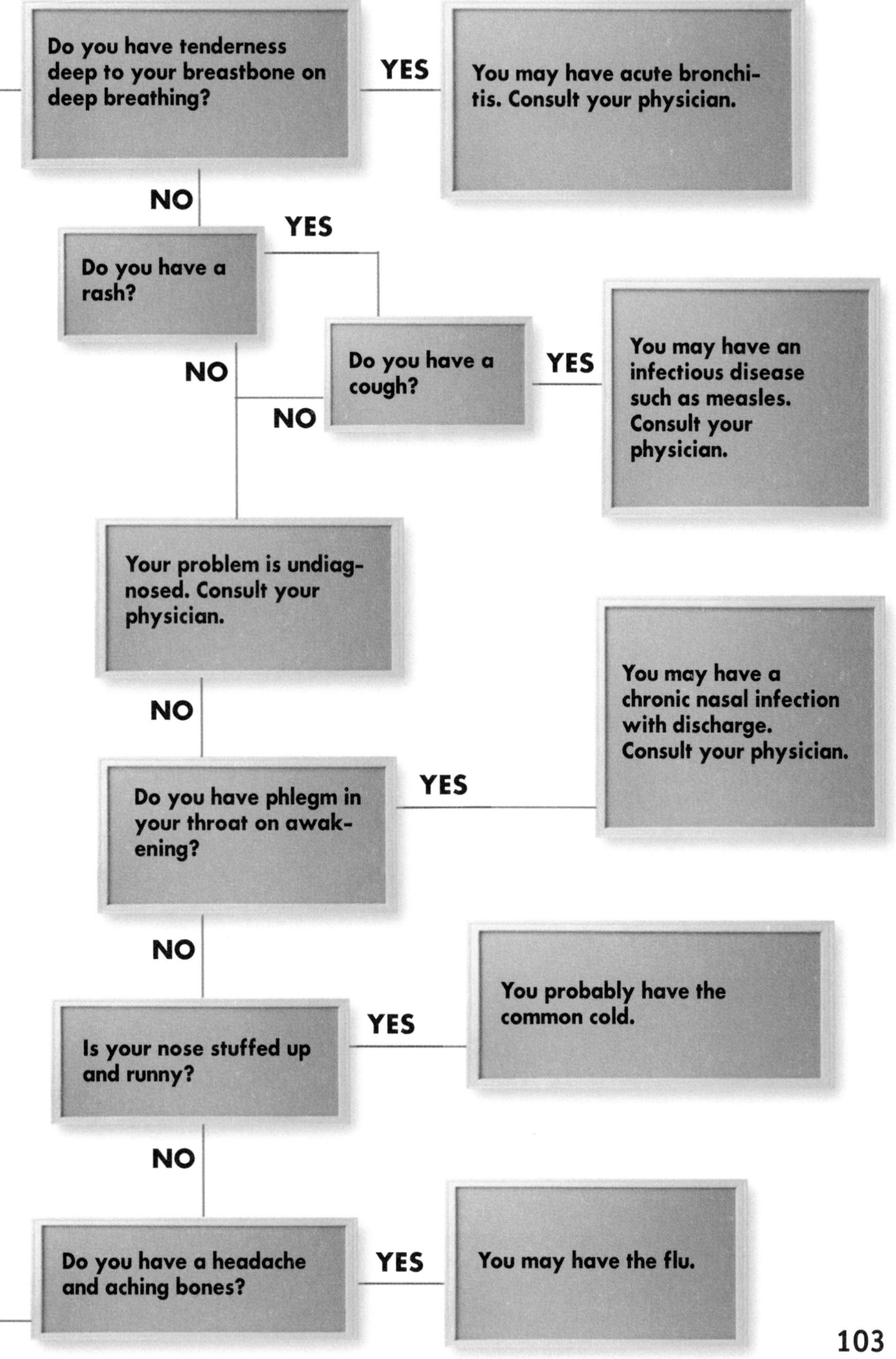
Do you have tenderness deep to your breastbone on deep breathing?
YES
You may have acute bronchitis. Consult your physician.
NO
Do you have a rash?
YES
NO
Do you have a cough?
YES
You may have an infectious disease such as measles. Consult your physician.
NO
Your problem is undiagnosed. Consult your physician.
NO
Do you have phlegm in your throat on awakening?
YES
You may have a chronic nasal infection with discharge. Consult your physician.
NO
Is your nose stuffed up and runny?
YES
You probably have the common cold.
NO
Do you have a headache and aching bones?
YES
You may have the flu.

Simple home treatments

Chapter Outline

- Applying heat and cold (thermotherapy)
- Hydrotherapy procedures
- Important considerations
- Applications of dry heat
- Sunbath
- Progressive relaxation

The human body—your body—is undoubtedly the most remarkable and intricate living "machine" in this world. If you are not familiar with the many systems that make up your body, it would be time well spent for you to become so. It will also be profitable for you to understand and practice simple measures you must take to preserve the efficient functioning of your body's systems. Living healthfully will enable you to keep your performance at top level for the longest period, and at the same time postpone the onset of disease and the frailties of old age.

But each person has a different background and has inherited a different constitution. We have also lived different lifestyles—either a lifestyle that has minimized the wear and tear of everyday living, or one that has neglected the principles of good maintenance. We have each been given a body that must last us a lifetime, and, sad to say, there are no trade-ins. There is just one per customer.

But the time comes, sooner or later, and sometimes sooner than later, when things go wrong. Structures wear out, inherited defects make their appearance, faulty health habits take their toll, our resistance drops, and we become sick. What should we do then? Call a physician? Rush to a hospital? The answer is Yes and No.

It would be ridiculous, if not impossible, for you to call a physician about every slight ache or pain. Reasonable people use simple remedies for the relief and cure of minor injuries and illnesses. Actually, the medical profession encourages such a practice. The average person is no

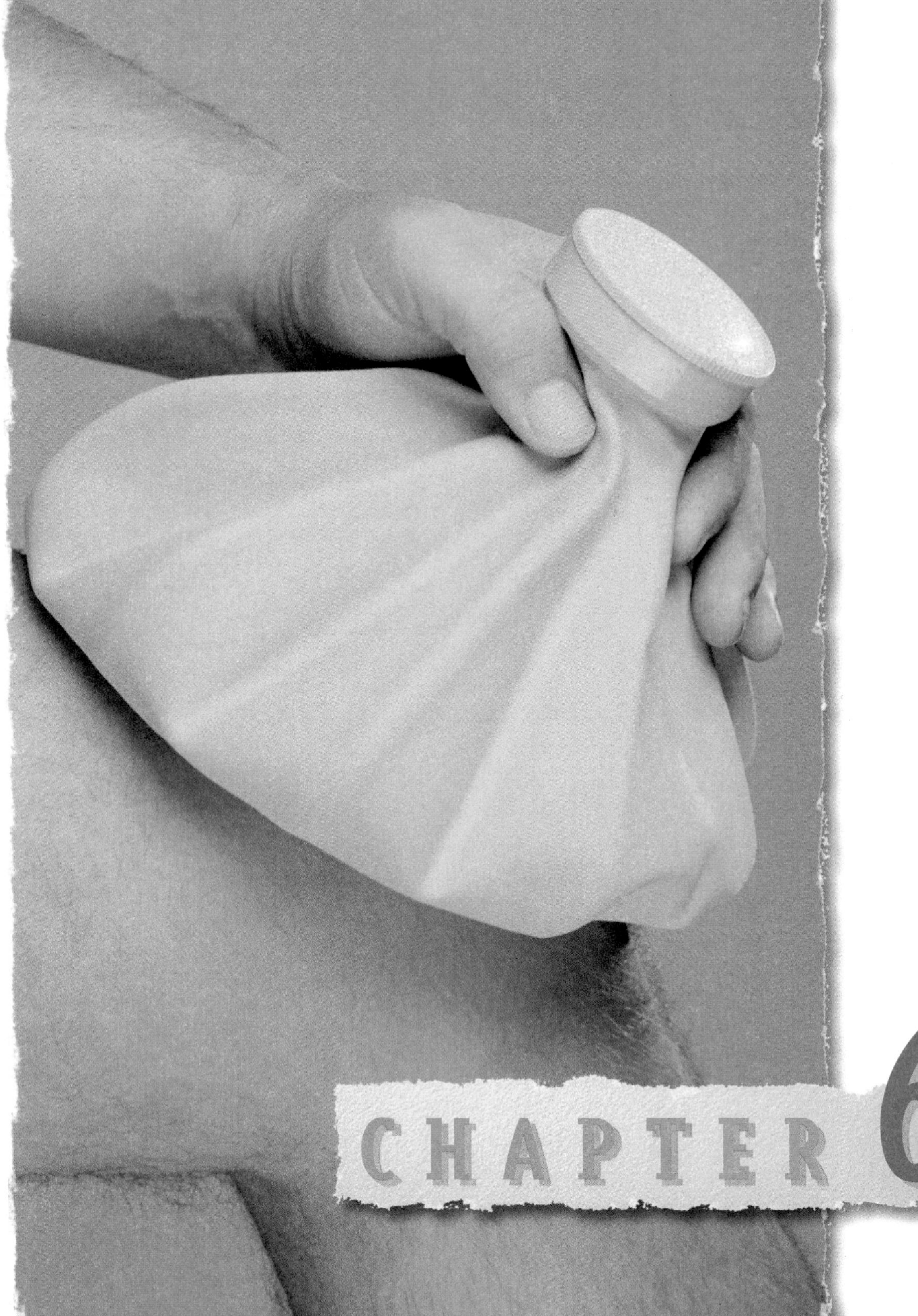

CHAPTER 6

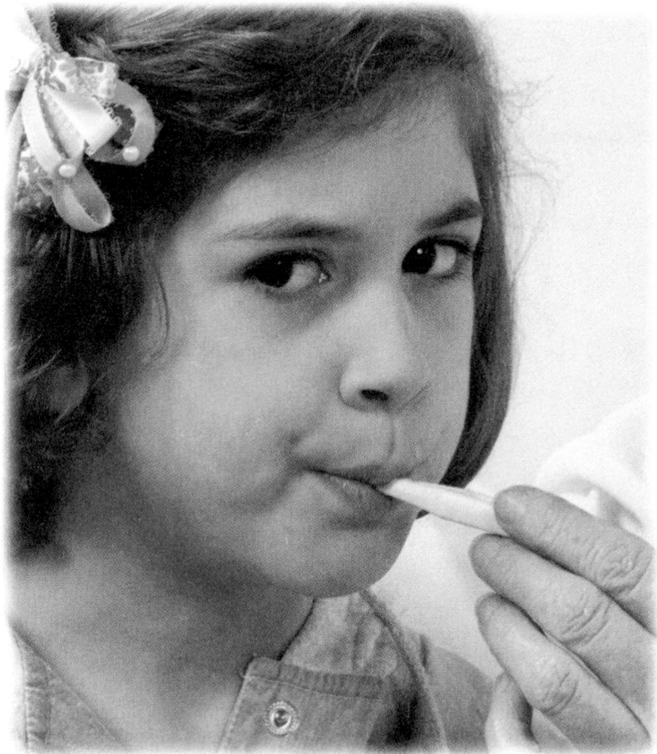

It would be ridiculous, if not impossible, for you to call a physician about every slight ache or pain.

more skilled in determining what is wrong with himself than he is in knowing what is wrong with his computer. However, just as there are a number of simple things you can do to solve computer problems, so there are several simple things you might do to solve illness problems.

The difficult decision is in knowing when to treat yourself and when to call a skilled professional. Here are a few suggestions that may prove helpful.

When to get medical help

You should always seek medical help, and not just use home treatments, under any of the following conditions:

- When a symptom is severe.
- When it persists.
- When it returns frequently.
- When you have any question as to its significance.
- When you are doubtful about what you are doing.

Unfortunately, the bathroom cabinets in many homes are stocked with medicines for headache, acid stomach, sleeplessness, and on and on, which family members use rather indiscriminately. Self-medication is encouraged by advertisements on television and radio, in the press, and in the drugstore. People are all too ready to take chemicals that provide temporary relief of the uncomfortable symptoms, while doing permanent damage to their bodies.

On the other hand, simple procedures and remedies that leave no harmful residual effects are available to everyone. These remedies make use of simple agencies such as water, light, controlled exercise, and rest. Their results depend on the body's natural response to its surroundings and to its own activity. While it is true that the use of these procedures should be restricted to minor ills, they often bring benefit with a relatively small expenditure of time and money, and without the harmful side effects of drugs and medications. Keep in mind that **any major treatment suggested in this book should be carried out with the approval of your physician.**

Readers who wish to become skilled in the use of the simple home procedures outlined in this chapter should take a course in these methods, or at least purchase a book about them. We especially recommend *Simple Remedies for the Home* by Clarence Dail and Charles Thomas, Preventive Health Care and Education Center, 4027 W. George Street, Banning, California 92220. The authors of this medical set drew heavily on the work of these men in writing this chapter.

Applying heat and cold (thermotherapy)

Skin and mucous membranes cover the structures (tissues and organs) that make up our bodies. However, these are much more than mere coverings. The skin and mucous membranes are equipped with detectors for heat, cold, touch, pressure, and pain. The skin also plays a major role in regulating the temperature of the body.

With few exceptions, the application of heat and cold as a medical treatment is made on the skin. As heat and cold pass through the skin (or mucous membrane), the temperatures of the underlying structures are altered, and ultimately the temperature of the body as a whole is affected.

The body is designed to maintain the equilibrium of its various systems. That is, it resists changes in temperature or any of its other myriad functions. This resistance to change is called *homeostasis*. However, you can stimulate chemical and physiological changes by applying heat and cold, and often as heat and cold penetrate the tissues, they have a healing effect. In addition, through nerve connections, reactions to heat and cold in the skin may reflexively affect organs deep within the body, initiating responses that are favorable to recovery.

Sources of heat and cold

Heat and cold can be applied to the body in a number of ways. The most common sources are water (hot or cold), infrared lamp or heater, sunshine, and things as simple as a heating pad or hot-water

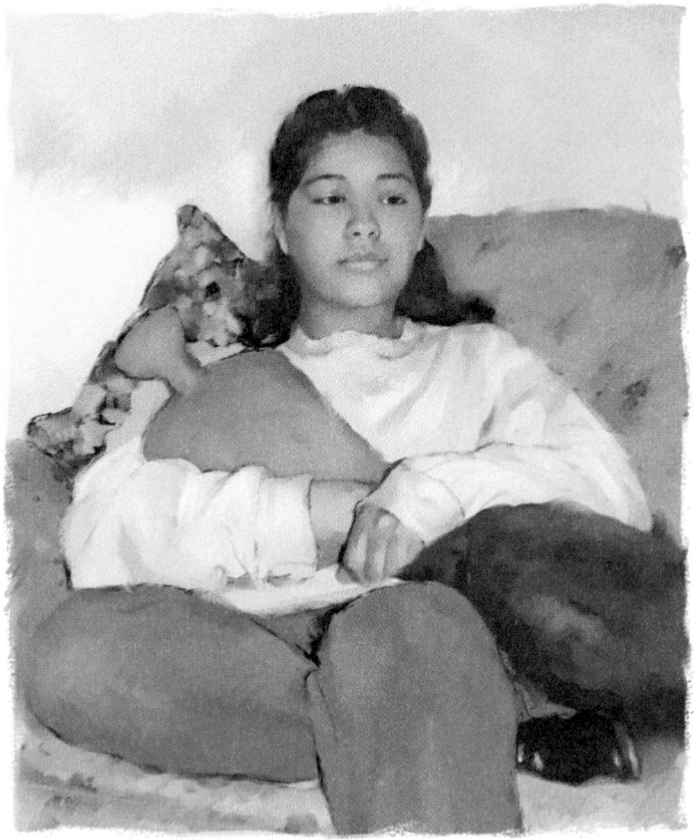

Alternating heat and cold generally increases local circulation.

bottle. Heat and cold enter or leave the body by radiation, conduction, convection, evaporation, and friction. The application of heat and cold can be wet, such as a hot foot bath, hot shower, steam inhalation, alcohol rub, or cold shower; or the application may be dry, as with a heat lamp, electric-light cabinet, sunshine, or an ice pack.

Effects of heat and cold

The application of heat and cold affects the circulation of the blood. It also causes certain chemical responses to occur within the blood and produces a number of chemical responses within the affected tissues.

Heat dilates blood vessels and increases the circulation of blood, both in the local area where the heat is applied and, in general, throughout the body. It also increases the congestion (accumulation) of blood near the skin and decreases its congestion deeper within the body. It accelerates the clotting of blood and increases white blood cell activity (phagocytosis). Heat warms local tissues and the whole body and increases swelling in the area where it is applied by drawing blood and tissue fluids into the area. Finally, heat increases glandular activity and muscular relaxation, and stimulates the body's chemical and physiological activity.

For the most part, the effects of **cold** are the opposite of those caused by heat. The blood vessels constrict, local and general circulation slows down, and congestion (accumulation) of blood deeper within the body is increased. Blood clotting is prolonged, and white cell activity decreases. The body as a whole is cooled, swelling in local tissues is diminished, muscles contract, and chemical and physiological activities are slowed down.

Alternating heat and cold generally increases local circulation, increases white blood cell activity, probably accelerates the clotting of blood, constricts blood vessels, and increases muscular activity.

With this understanding of the

effects of heat and cold, we can make applications in specific ways to help the body's recovery processes. For example, immediately after a person has sprained his ankle, the application of cold will cause the flow of blood and other tissue fluids through the area to diminish, thus helping to keep the swelling down.

Breathing warm, moist air from a steam inhalator helps to relieve throat irritation and loosens secretions in the trachea and bronchi. It soothes the inflamed membranes, and, interestingly, at first facilitates coughing, but later relieves it.

Most of these effects are due to the direct action of either heating or cooling the tissues. However, as already mentioned, the body resists changes that tend to upset its normal equilibrium (homeostasis). It tries to prevent change by doing things that react against it. For example, sweating is one of the body's common reactions to heat, which is the body's effort to stay cool. On the other hand, shivering is a typical reaction to cold—the body's effort to stay warm. The body's reaction to heat may produce a sedative effect in the patient, as with a warm bath; its reaction to cold may be tonic, as with a short, cold shower. The desired effect is obtained by applying heat and cold in the right way. It is therefore important that hot and cold treatments be given properly.

Hydrotherapy procedures

Hot foot bath

The hot foot bath is one of the most useful of all water treatments. It is simple to do and produces several beneficial effects. The blood flow is increased locally, and if the foot bath is prolonged, there is general warming and increased blood flow in distant parts of the body. Congestion in the pelvic organs, chest, and head is decreased.

Uses. A number of conditions are benefited. These include a head cold, sore throat, cough, and bronchitis. Cramps in the pelvic organs may be relieved, as well as headache. There is generalized muscular relaxation. It is quite effective for nosebleed.

Contraindications. Do not apply heat to the feet or legs in any condition in which the circulation is poor, such as diabetes, atherosclerosis of the lower limbs, and diseases of the peripheral blood vessels. Nor should heat be applied to the feet or legs when there is acute swelling from a sprain or arthritis, loss of feeling in the legs and feet, or when the patient is unconscious.

Procedure. Use a container (plastic or metal) sufficiently large

Testing the temperature of water to be used in treatment should be done with a thermometer as well as with the hand.

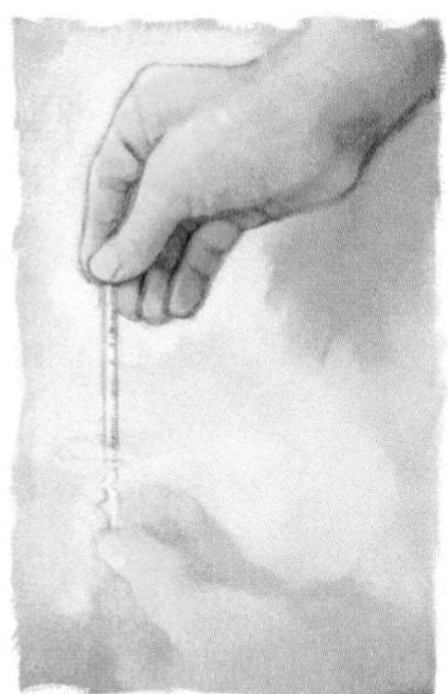

Important considerations

Heat and *cold* are comparative terms and must be defined. This, unfortunately, cannot be done with accuracy, since people differ in their tolerance to heat and cold. The temperature sensation produced by water varies according to the condition of the skin, its previous temperature, the vigor of blood circulation, and even the season of the year. Testing the temperature of water to be used in treatment, therefore, should be done *with a thermometer* as well as with the hand.

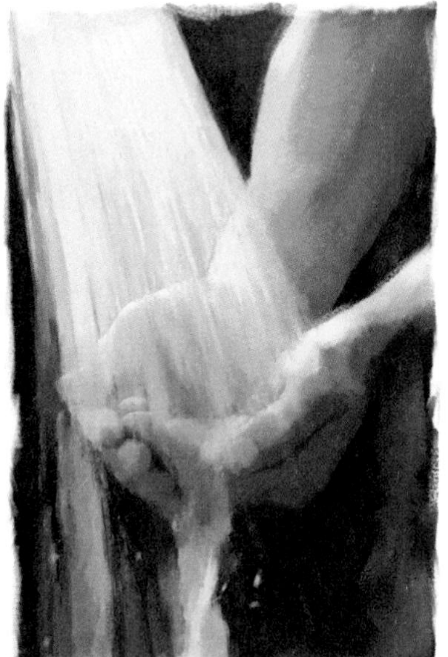

When applying heat and cold, great care must be exercised to avoid damage to the skin and underlying tissues. Patients must not be chilled or overheated, nor, of course, should they be burned.

Careful, thoughtful consideration must be given as to what the particular procedure will do to the patient. Take, for example, the case of a diabetic with atherosclerosis to whom you are considering giving a hot foot bath. Locally applied heat increases the tissue's need for oxygen, and therefore for more blood. The fact that he has atherosclerosis may mean that the circulation in his feet is impaired, limiting the amount of blood that can be drawn to his feet should heat be applied. Giving a hot foot bath to such an individual would increase the demand for oxygen and for increased blood flow. Since it may not be possible to provide sufficient blood, tissue damage is likely to occur, and even gangrene may be precipitated.

The treatments described on the following pages use water and other simple means. Note the different uses and precautions (contraindications—when not to use a procedure), and follow the directions carefully.

to accommodate the feet, that will allow water to cover the ankles. The water temperature should range between 104 and 112°F (40 to 44°C). Begin the treatment at a lower temperature, and periodically add hot water, thus gradually increasing the bath temperature according to the tolerance of the patient. The treatment should last ten to fifteen minutes. Encourage the drinking of cool or warm water. Be sure to place your hand between the hot water and the patient's feet any time you pour more hot water into the container.

The treatment can be given while the patient is lying in bed (bedclothes should be protected with a plastic) or while he is sitting in a chair. Small children can place their feet in a kitchen sink. Keep the upper body warm with a light blanket or large bath towel. Apply a cold compress to the patient's head, and replace it every two or three minutes. When the treatment is over, lift the feet out of the water, pour cold water over them, and dry them thoroughly. Should the patient be sweating generally, dry him with a towel, followed by an alcohol rub. Let the patient rest, lightly covered, for about twenty minutes before getting up.

Hot-and-cold immersion baths (for arm/hand and leg/foot)

In this treatment, a part of the patient's body is alternately immersed in hot and then cold water. This increases the circulation in the area, first causing dilation of the blood vessels, then contraction. Swelling is reduced, and phagocytic activity (destruction of foreign microorganisms by white blood cells) is increased.

Uses. Similar to those of a hot foot bath, but also very effective in reducing the swelling from a sprained ankle or wrist, twenty-four hours after the accident occurred. (Initially a cold compress or cold foot bath is indicated.) It is also useful for an infection in the extremities.

Contraindications. Similar contraindications as for a hot footbath, but not as stringent.

Procedure. Obtain plastic or metal containers sufficiently large and deep to immerse a foot and leg or a hand and arm. Fill one with hot water (see hot foot bath), and the other with cold or ice water. Place the patient's foot and leg into the hot water (as hot as can be tolerated without burning) for three minutes, then plunge it into the cold water for thirty seconds.

While the limb is in the cold water, pour additional hot water into the hot tub to maintain or raise the temperature, taking care not to make it so hot that it will burn the patient. This should be done four or five times for a complete treatment. A towel should be handy to dry the extremity, which should not be allowed to chill. Often the heat

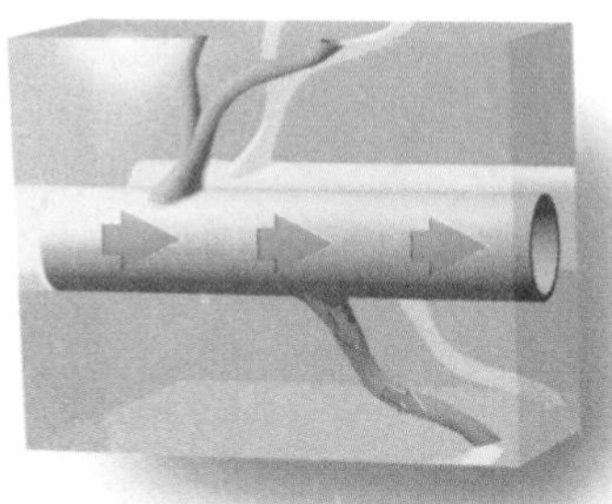

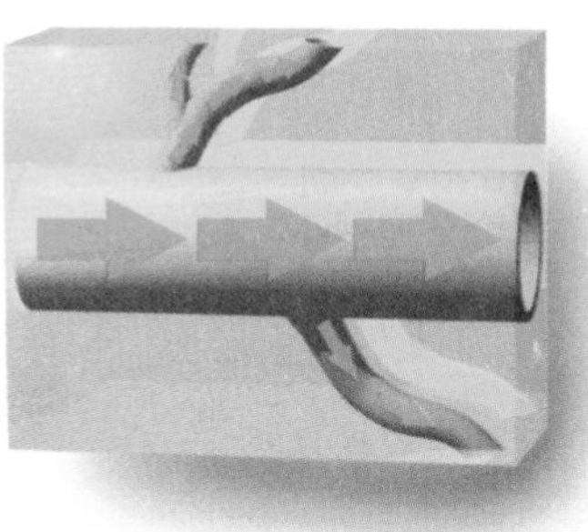

The application of cold will cause the flow of blood and other tissue fluids through the area to diminish, thus helping to keep the swelling down. The application of heat will have the opposite effect.

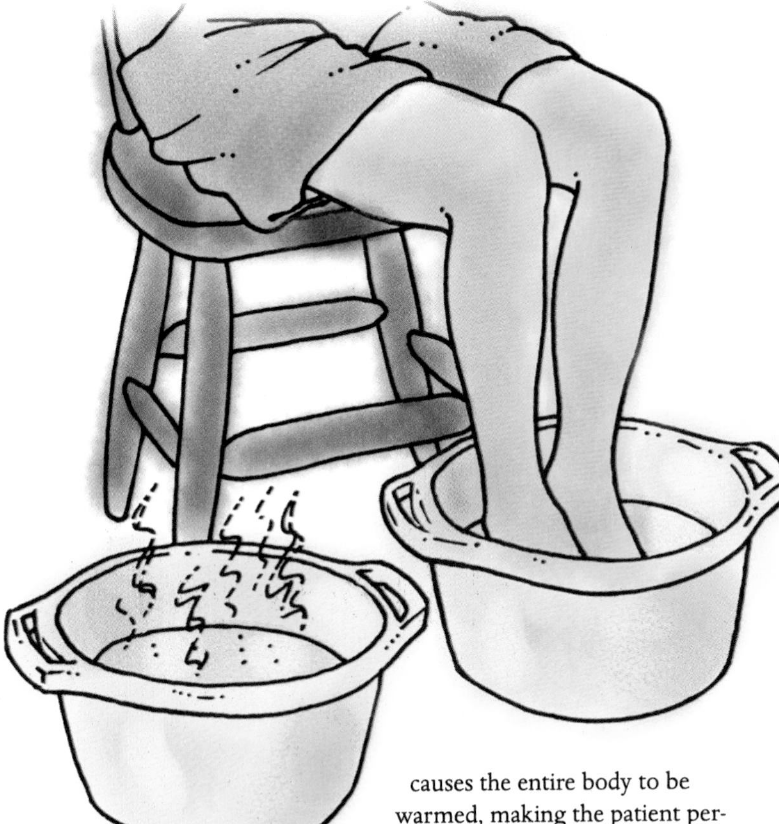

Hot and cold leg and foot bath.

causes the entire body to be warmed, making the patient perspire. If this begins to happen, apply a cold compress to the forehead during the treatment. When the procedure is complete, the patient may take a warm shower and dry off, or, if he is in bed, he can be dried off and have a brisk alcohol rub.

Fomentations

A fomentation is the application of moist heat to some area of the skin by means of a heated, moistened cloth pad. This localized, sudden application of heat increases surface blood flow, relieves internal congestion, increases the circulation of white blood cells, relieves muscle spasm and certain types of pain, promotes sweating, and causes generalized relaxation.

Uses. Fomentations are often helpful for the common cold, coughs, bronchitis, and influenza. They also provide relief from the pain of neuralgia and certain forms of arthritis. Applied to the spine (warm, not hot), fomentations produce sedation and help to combat insomnia.

Contraindications. Do not apply fomentations to the limbs of those with peripheral vascular disorders or to diabetics. Neither should fomentations be used on an unconscious or paralyzed person. If given to a patient who has recently had a heart attack, check with his physician first, and if administered, place an ice bag over the heart.

Procedure. The fomentation pad is best made of blanket material that consists of 50 percent wool to retain heat and 50 percent cotton to hold water. A thick Turkish towel or thick terry cloth may also be used. Six pads are made from cut material, 30 x 36 inches (75 x 90 cm), folded in thirds, and then sewn so that the finished pad is 12 x 30 inches (30 x 75 cm). Have available some eight to ten light, medium-sized towels, two large bath towels, four washcloths, and a bowl of ice water.

The pads may be heated in one of three ways: (1) Fold a pad in thirds and twist it into a loose roll. Holding the two ends, immerse the middle portion in a large kettle of boiling water. Then pull the ends, twisting at the same time to wring the pad as dry as possible. (2) Moisten the pads and place them in a steam boiler (not in water) until they are thoroughly heated. (3) Place moistened pads in a microwave oven until they are heated. This is the most convenient method.

When the heated pad is wrung dry or removed from the steamer or microwave oven, wrap it in a light towel, fold it double, and roll it up to retain the heat. You may make three of these heated rolled-up pads in quick succession.

Before beginning the treatment, see that the room is comfortably warm. It is extremely important that the patient not be chilled at any time. Have the patient disrobe and lie down. Place a large bath towel underneath and another over the patient, then cover him with a blanket. Place a light towel over the area to which the hot fomentation pad is to be applied—the chest, for example. Place a heated fomentation cloth on the towel covering the chest. A few moments later lift one side of the pad and then the other, and wipe the chest with a dry face cloth to prevent burning. If the pad is too hot, place an additional light towel between the pad and the patient.

Place extra coverings (face cloths), if needed, over bony prominences or the nipples, lest they burn.

As soon as the patient is reasonably comfortable, place the second fomentation underneath him, lengthwise along the spine. Then wrap one around the feet, unless contraindicated, and wrap it in a towel. This may be done in place of a hot foot bath.

Prepare additional hot fomentations to replace the one on the chest every three to five minutes three in all. Fomentations should be tolera-

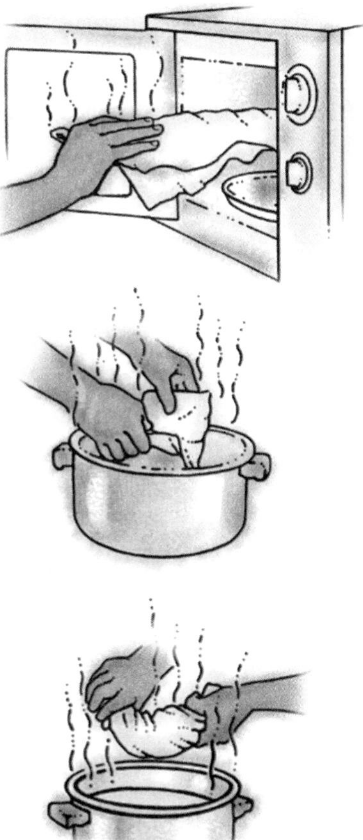

Three ways of preparing fomentation cloths: (1) heating damp cloths in a microwave oven; (2)steaming moistened cloths in a kettle; (3) dipping cloths in hot water.

ble but not necessarily comfortable. Before replacing a fomentation pad, dry the heated skin quickly. (Removing the moisture remaining on the skin makes it easier to endure the heat of the newly prepared fomentation.) A fresh, dry, light towel should replace the one on the skin each time a fomentation pad is changed. Fomentations on the spine and feet are not changed.

Keep a cold, folded, wet face cloth on the forehead during the procedure, recooling it frequently. Allow the patient to drink as much cool water as he desires through a bent straw. After the fomentation is removed the last time, wipe the skin briskly with a cold, wet facecloth. Dry the patient immediately, and cover him with a blanket to prevent chilling. Following the complete treatment, allow the patient to lie quietly for at least thirty minutes.

Hot and cold to the chest

This application is similar to the fomentation, with one important modification.

Uses. Aids in the treatment of chest colds, coughs, and bronchitis. Stimulates deep breathing.

Contraindications. These include: recent surgery, malignancy, pleurisy, impaired sensation, and impaired circulation. Also excluded are children under twelve, and patients who are paralyzed or unconscious.

Procedure. Start a fomentation to the chest as described above. When the fomentation is removed, dry the chest immediately. Have the patient take a deep breath, and rub his chest briskly with ice, covering the area twice. This should be done at the end of each chest fomentation. Otherwise follow the routine for fomentations.

Cold mitten friction

With this procedure, cold is rapidly applied section by section to the skin, using cold wet face cloths or cold wet mitts.

Uses. Cold mitten friction builds resistance to cold as well as general body resistance. Phagocytic action is increased, as is antibody production. This treatment stimulates the circulation and is useful in terminating a fomentation. It can also be used to end the morning shower.

Contraindications. Do not use this procedure when the patient is chilled, nor should friction be applied to skin lesions or eruptions.

Procedure. A face cloth that has been folded in half and sewed on two sides makes an excellent bag or mitt into which the hand can be placed. The patient should be warm, undressed, and lying between two light blankets or large bath towels. Dip the mitt in cold water, wring out any excess water, and put it on your hands. Start with the extremities, then the chest, and finally the back. Vigorously rub the skin of one arm for five to eight seconds. Dry the arm immediately, and cover it to keep it warm. Follow with the other arm, then the lower extremities, and finally the chest and back. Apply a cold compress to the forehead during the procedure.

Hot mitten friction

The method of application is similar to that of cold mitten friction, except that hot water is used instead of cold. This procedure is excellent for warming a chilled patient and for producing relaxation and inducing sleep. Do not apply this treatment on skin lesions or to an overheated patient.

Cold compress

A cold compress is a cold or ice cold wet cloth applied to some part of the body. It decreases the local flow of blood, prevents congestion in a limited area, and relieves pain due to swelling or injury. When applied over the heart, it slows the rate of the heartbeat.

Uses. A cold compress lessens the pain and swelling of a sprain of the wrist or ankle when applied immediately after the injury has occurred. It relieves sinus congestion and

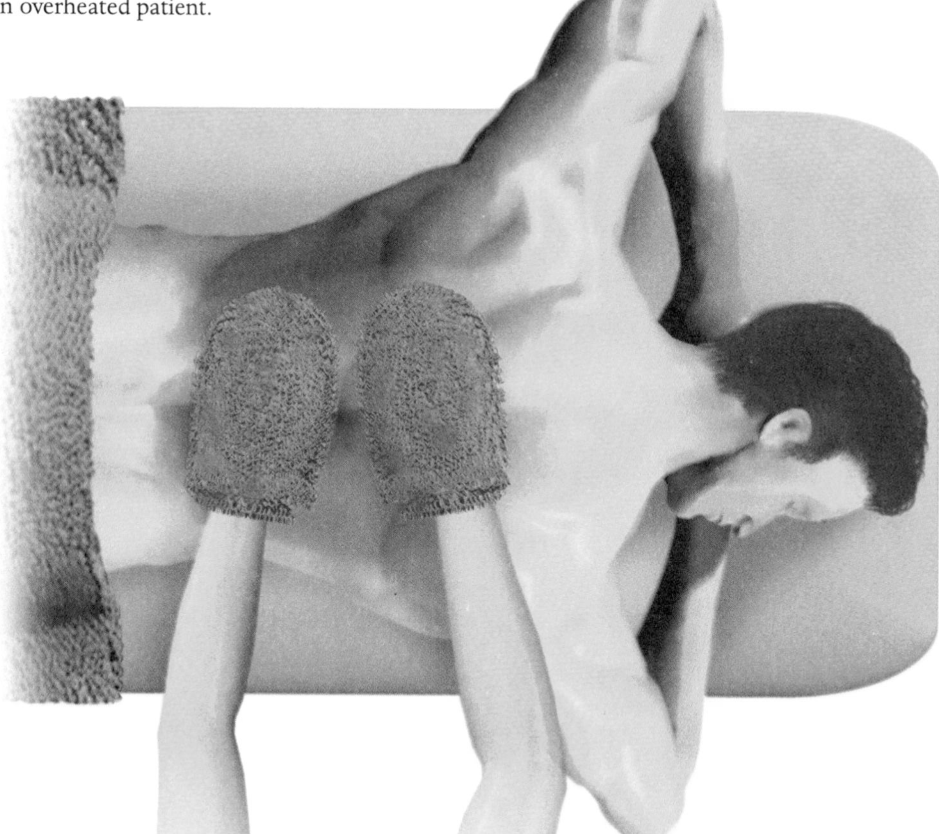

Rapidly apply cold to the skin, section by section, using cold, wet face cloths, or cold, wet mitts.

headaches, slows the heart rate in tachycardia, and provides relief when applied to the forehead during fever, or when general body warming procedures are being employed.

Contraindications. Cold compresses should not be used on patients with diabetes, skin diseases, or those who have an intolerance to cold or who are chilled.

Procedure. Use an ordinary small hand towel or face cloth, fold it to the desired size, and wet it in cold or ice water. Wring out the water just enough so that it does not drip. Renew every two to five minutes. Apply the compress firmly to the patient's forehead, ankle, heart, or wherever desired. Be sure the patient is warm before starting the treatment.

Warm, moist air rising from a pan of hot water may be inhaled, reducing congestion.

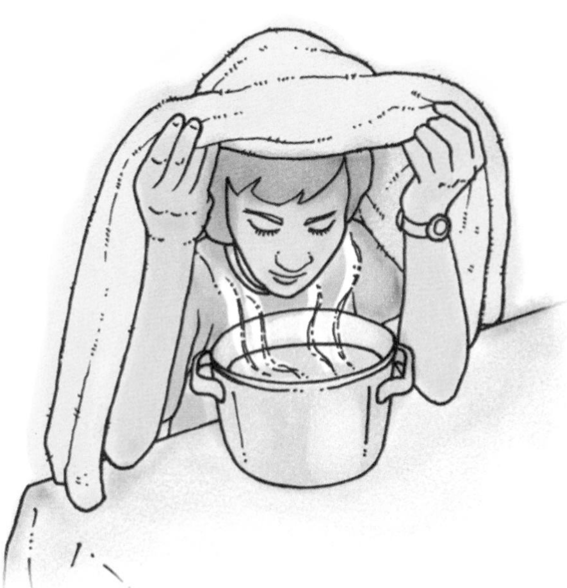

Heating compress

A wet heating compress is a cold, wet, lightweight cloth or several layers of wet gauze applied to a localized area of the body, covered with a wool (or similar material) bandage, and held in place for several hours, allowing the body to first warm and later dry the compress. It initially produces constriction of the blood vessels, followed by dilation. Depending on the location and size of the compress, it may produce general warming and sweating.

Uses. The wet heating compress helps to relieve the pain of acute sore throat (pharyngitis, laryngitis, tonsillitis), joint pain from arthritis and rheumatic fever, chest cold, cough, chronic bronchitis, and asthma. For pleurisy, use a "dry" heating compress.

Contraindications. Do not use this procedure if the patient is unable to warm up the compress (may use a heat lamp or hot-water bottle to facilitate warming). Do not allow chilling. If chilling seems likely, discontinue the procedure and use a "dry" heating compress instead.

Procedure. Heating compresses can be applied to the neck, ankle, wrists, and other desired parts. Dip a piece of cotton cloth in cold water and wring it dry. Quickly place the cloth around the desired area, wrap it with a wool (or similar) bandage, fastening it with safety pins. Allow it to remain in place for several hours or overnight. On removal, wipe the area with a cool, damp cloth, then dry thoroughly.

The strip of wool cloth should be 3 to 4 inches wide (7.5 to 12 cm) and about 6 inches (15 cm) longer than the cotton cloth strip. The width and length of the bandages are determined by their use. For a neck compress, the cloth strip should be about 3 x 30 inches (7.5 x 75 cm), while the wool strip should be about 4 x 36 inches (12 x 90 cm). For the chest, the strips should be proportionately wider and longer. Always see that the cold wet strip is well covered by the dry wool cloth.

The method for using a dry heating compress is identical to that of the wet heating compress, except that the thin cotton cloth is not wet, but is applied dry. For example, if a dry heating compress is to be applied to the chest, a thin cotton undershirt can be worn and covered with a long sleeved wool sweater.

Steam inhalation

This application provides warm, moist air to the respiratory passageways that relieves inflammation and congestion, loosens secretions, prompts discharge from the throat and lungs, and prevents drying of the respiratory membranes.

Uses. Steam inhalation relieves coughing and congestion of the nose, throat, and bronchi. It loosens dry and thick secretions in the airways, and soothes a dry, irritated throat.

Contraindications. Infants, very young children, and the very aged may not be able to handle the heat.

Procedure. There are a number of ways in which moist, warm air can be provided to a patient. Commercial steam inhalators are available at moderate expense and are very convenient. Directions require filling a small container with water and plugging in the device. In a few minutes steam is projected through a small aperture. Most brands will function continuously for eight or more hours. The inhalator can be placed on the floor or on a stool near the head of the bed. Children should not be able to reach the inhalator, as steam may burn their hands. The patient does not need to be placed in a tent.

If you do not have access to a commercial inhalator, you can boil water on the kitchen stove and inhale the steam (beware of burns from getting too close to the boiling water), or boil water in a teakettle on an electric portable burner in the bedroom. If concentrated steam is desired, the steam from the inhalator or kettle can be directed toward the patient with a newspaper that has been rolled into a cone shape. Another way to concentrate the warm vapor is to erect a "tent" over the bed with a sheet and allow the steam to flow into the tent.

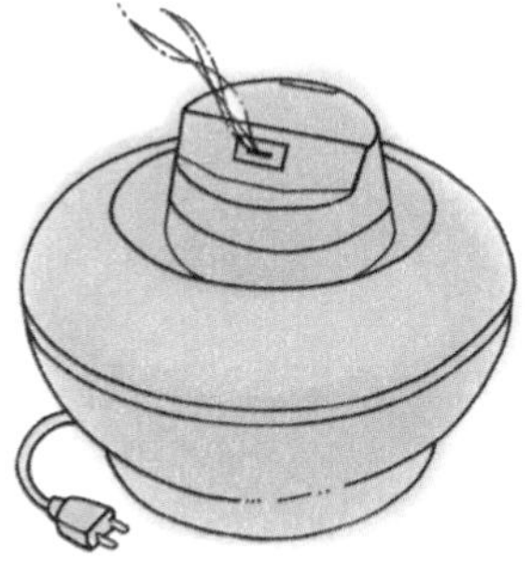

Warm, moist air from a commercial vaporizer soothes the respiratory passageways.

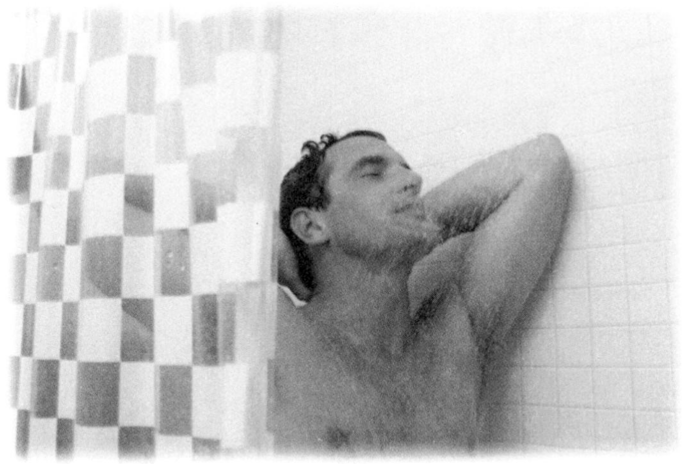

Hot and cold waters are stimulating.

You can medicate the water with a few drops of pine oil or eucalyptus oil. However, remember that some people are allergic to these oils, especially to pine oil.

Showers

A shower is a device by which multiple small streams of water are directed under pressure onto some surface of the body. It is one of the cheapest and best forms of home therapy. Depending on the temperature of the water, a shower can be relaxing or stimulating, warming or cooling. It can improve the general circulation. It can be used for ambulatory patients, and even for those who can sit while the shower is running.

Uses. A shower will relieve the pain from bruises and muscle spasms. It can warm a chilled person or preheat for a cold application, such as a cold shower. It is refreshing and cleansing. The common cold and bronchitis are helped.

Contraindications. Persons with heart disease, advanced atherosclerosis, certain kidney diseases, high blood pressure, and hyperthyroidism should avoid showers. A cold shower is especially not suitable for a rheumatic patient.

Procedure. A shower can be taken in a number of ways. If a person is chilled, a warm to hot shower will produce general warming. Hot and cold showers are stimulating. Bring the water to body temperature for a minute or so before ending the shower. Gradually increase the temperature to tolerance, and then abruptly turn the hot water off, allowing the cold water to strike the skin for about ten seconds. Over time, healthy people can learn to tolerate cold for longer and longer periods. Some like to take a hot shower and end by giving a cold mitten friction. Plain cold showers can be used for their stimulating action.

Precautions. Have a stool available in case the patient should feel faint. Care should be taken that the patient does not slip or fall. Do not allow the patient to become chilled after a shower.

Tub bath

Immersing the entire body in water is a simple but effective means of altering the function of major body systems. A **hot tub bath** increases the general circulation, raises body temperature, and is relaxing. A **graduated tub bath** is effective in lowering body temperature. A **neutral bath** is calming.

Uses. A hot bath improves the general circulation, relieving the congestion of the internal organs. Also, it alleviates stiffness and pain in the muscles and lessens fatigue. A graduated bath is effective in lowering elevated body temperature, as in a fever. A neutral bath aids in calming an agitated patient and relieves nervous tension.

Contraindications. People with heart and valvular diseases, vascular disorders, high blood pressure, diabetes, and cancers should avoid hot tub baths. Also, elderly and frail persons do not tolerate a hot bath.

Procedure. For a **hot tub bath**, obtain the consent of the patient's physician. The tub should be two-thirds full of water at about 101 to 103°F (38 to 39.5°C). Assist the patient into the tub. Have him lie down so that water covers his chest. Place a cold compress on his forehead and cover his knees (if they are exposed above the water) with a towel. Encourage him to drink a glass of water. The initial bath should be no longer than ten minutes, with a rise in body temperature of no more than one degree. If well tolerated, subsequent baths can be longer (not to exceed twenty minutes), with water temperature somewhat higher (not to exceed 106°F. (41°C]). Patients should be watched closely, as they sometimes feel faint. Following the bath, dry the skin thoroughly, and finish with an alcohol rub or a cool sponge. During the treatment take the patient's pulse and temperature at five-minute intervals.

For a **graduated bath**, commence with a water temperature of approximately 100°F (38°C). Maintain this temperature for three minutes, then gradually lower the temperature with cold water to about 94°F (34°C)over a period of five minutes. If the patient tolerates the cooler water, gradually lower the temperature to 90°F (32°C). If the patient feels chilly or develops goose pimples, rub his skin constantly with a face cloth. Do not allow him to become chilled. At the end of the bath, dry the patient promptly and thoroughly, and wrap him in a warm blanket.

For a **neutral bath**, maintain the water temperature at slightly below normal body temperature—approximately 97°F (36°C)—for at least twenty to thirty minutes, longer if well tolerated. Do not allow the patient to chill. Keep the room warm. Following the bath, dry the patient thoroughly but avoid unnecessary rubbing. Do not excite the patient as this destroys the sedative effect. Have the patient rest in bed following the bath for at least thirty minutes.

In a hot half-bath the person sits in the tub with water covering the legs, hips, and lower trunk.

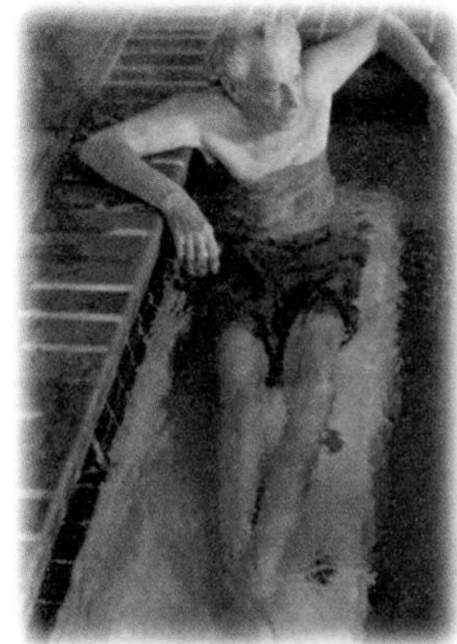

Hot half-bath

The person sits in the tub with water covering the legs, hips, and lower trunk. Blood is drawn from the upper to the lower body, and from the internal organs to the skin.

Uses. This procedure relieves congestion in the bronchi and sinuses, and pain in the low back and pelvic area. It may be used to raise the body temperature (artificial fever). Higher water temperatures can be tolerated than in a full tub bath since only part of the body is submerged.

Contraindications. Avoid this procedure on patients who have heart disease, diabetes, and atherosclerosis, especially of the legs and feet.

Procedure. The person sits in a tub of water that has been heated initially to 101°F (38°C). Cover his legs, hips, and lower trunk. Gradually raise the temperature of the water by adding hot water and removing tub water. The water temperature should be raised to tolerance, not to exceed 112°F (44°C). The bath should last from five to twenty minutes. Apply a cold compress to the forehead and drape a towel over the exposed shoulders. The bath may be ended by dashing a pail of cold water over the lower body and limbs, or by using a cold sponge. Dry the patient promptly. When the patient first stands up, watch closely for possible fainting. Take his pulse and mouth temperature at five-minute intervals.

The **sitz bath** is a version of the hot half-bath in which the patient sits in a tub of hot water with his feet outside, placed in a hot footbath. The water in the tub should cover the patient's hips. Higher water temperatures can be maintained in the pelvic area without causing as much general heating of the body. The other procedures are similar to those described under the hot half-bath. It has been used effectively in relieving menstrual cramps and in treating (or as an adjunct treatment) for inflammatory conditions of the pelvis.

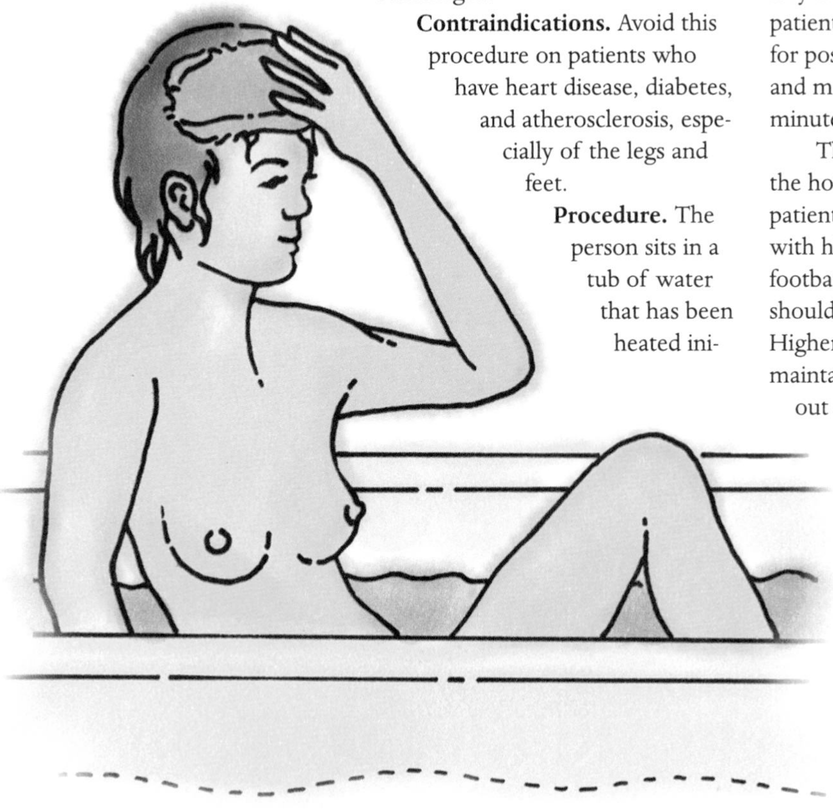

A hot half-bath may be taken in a bathtub. Note the cold compress to the forehead.

Ice water or ice pack

The application of ice water or an ice pack to a local area or to parts of a limb causes the contraction of blood vessels, slows down the oozing of blood, and prevents edema.

Uses. This procedure diminishes the swelling from bruises and sprains and also gives relief in conditions such as rheumatic fever, rheumatoid arthritis, and acute infectious arthritis. Ice water or an ice pack will also lessen the pain of acute bursitis and the pain from an inflamed joint. The pain and swelling of a small burn are reduced when cold water is applied immediately after the burn has occurred.

Procedure. Commercially made ice bags are available from a pharmacy, and are both convenient and effective. However, the following method can be successfully used. Spread crushed ice over a towel or piece of flannel so that it makes a 1-foot square (30 x 30 cm) of ice 1 inch deep (2.5 cm). The towel or cloth should be folded and safety pinned to hold the ice in place. Place the ice bag (or the towel or flannel containing the ice) on the part to be treated. Cover the area with plastic, then a towel. *Check periodically to avoid tissue injury. Do not let melted ice water soak onto the skin.* If well tolerated, the pack may be held in place with a bandage. The application may be continued up to thirty minutes. Remove the pack, dry the patient thoroughly, and cover him to keep warm.

Immediately following the spraining of an ankle or wrist, the injured joint may be gradually submerged in a bucket of cold or ice cold water. If the patient complains of the water being too cold, remove the limb momentarily and resubmerge it. The application may be continued for up to thirty minutes, depending on the patient's tolerance. These applications can be made for thirty minutes out of every two hours for up to six treatments.

Immediately following the spraining of an ankle or wrist, the injured joint may be gradually submerged in a bucket of cold or ice cold water.

For a small burn (finger, hand, etc.) place the affected area under cold running tap water or submerge it in a pan of ice cold water. Allow it to remain in the cold water until the pain is relieved, or for thirty minutes.

Sponge or rub

Sponging consists of applying water with a sponge, washcloth, or the bare hand, with little if any friction. A treatment in which water or

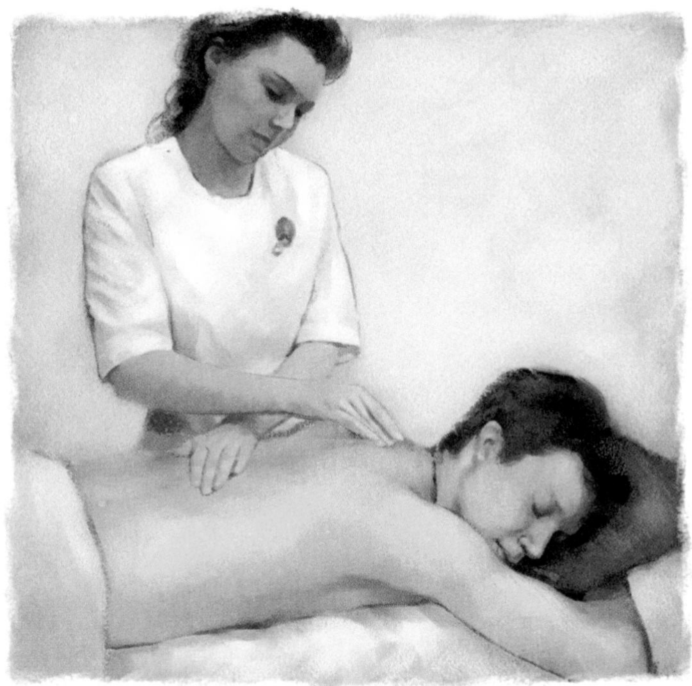

When rubbing alcohol is applied to the skin with the hand, it evaporates rapidly and lowers the body temperature.

some other liquid (lotion or cream) is applied with the bare hand is called a "rub," although little actual rubbing is done.

Uses. This treatment moistens the skin, soothes the patient, lowers body temperature, and reduces fever.

Procedure. Generally a washcloth is used, dipped in cool, tepid, or warm water, and squeezed out enough to prevent dripping. Each part of the body is gone over lightly, back and forth, until it is perceptibly cooler. Each part is then dried lightly, not rubbed. Hot sponging is used in fevers where there is chilliness, the same methods being followed as with cool or tepid sponging, except that less water is applied. Keep the patient covered except for the part being sponged.

Alcohol rub

Rubbing alcohol is applied to the skin with the hand. Alcohol has a drying action on the skin, precipitating the protein in the superficial cells. It evaporates rapidly, thus lowering body temperature.

Uses. This application cools the body, lowers the temperature, and refreshes the patient. It also toughens the skin, and is especially useful when applied to pressure points to prevent bedsores. It is very effective in terminating warming procedures such as hot showers, fomentations, hot tub baths, etc.

Contraindications. Do not use this treatment on infants and small children because of absorption through the skin and lungs (vapors inhaled).

Procedure. Rubbing alcohol (isopropyl alcohol) can be purchased from a drugstore for this purpose. Wood alcohol (methyl alcohol) should never be used. Regular alcohol (ethyl alcohol) can be used but should be diluted to 70 percent. A small amount of rubbing alcohol is poured into the palm of the hand and quickly rubbed over a portion of the patient's skin. Use both hands, spreading the alcohol over the arms, legs, chest, abdomen, and back. Keep the patient covered except where the alcohol is being applied.

Applications of dry heat

Hot-water bottle

A hot-water bottle is a most useful article in the sick room. Its warmth can be applied to many parts of the body.

Uses. A hot-water bottle relaxes, warms, and relieves congestion and pains. It will produce relaxation and induce sleep. It can augment the heating action of a hot compress or fomentation.

Contraindications. Never use a hot-water bottle with patients who have impaired sensation, who are paralyzed or unconscious, or who have poor circulation.

Procedure. Fill the bottle to two-thirds full with hot but not boiling water. Screw the top on lightly and expel the air by squeezing the bottle until the water reaches the neck. The stopper should then be screwed tight and the bottle held upside down to check for leaks. Place the bottle in a bag made from flannel or Turkish toweling and position it on the desired area of the patient. Never use an unprotected hot-water bottle.

Electric heating pad

The uses and contraindications of a heating pad are similar to those of a hot-water bottle. Pads come with a temperature range—mild, moderate, or high heat.

Radiant heat

Radiant heat is long infrared waves emanating from a heat source such as an electric heater, wood stove, or heat lamp. The waves strike the skin, warming it, and the heat gradually penetrates to the deeper tissues.

Uses. Heating pad treatments are similar to those of a hot-water bottle. In many cases, radiant heat benefits sufferers with neuralgia, neuritis, arthritis, and sinusitis.

Contraindications. Same as those for a hot-water bottle.

Procedure. Radiant heaters can be purchased from a medical supply store. However, an electric bathroom heater without a fan is an excellent source, as is an infrared bulb, available in most department stores. Heat can be applied for thirty minutes or longer, taking care to place the device at an appropriate distance from the part of the patient being treated. Do not overheat, as this may cause burns.

A hot-water bottle is a most useful article in the sick room. Its warmth can be applied to many parts of the body.

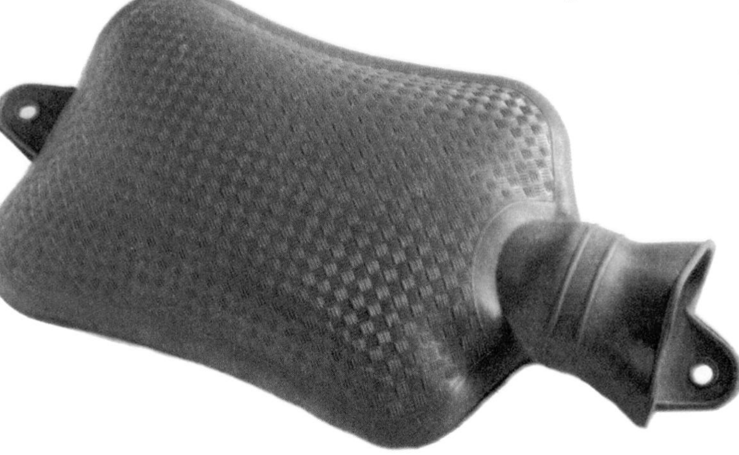

Sun bath

In a sun bath, areas of the skin are exposed to the direct rays of the sun.

In a sun bath, areas of the skin are exposed to the direct rays of the sun (solar radiation) for varying lengths of time. The three types of light waves ultraviolet, visible, and infrared—all have different effects on the skin and body as a whole. The skin may be either benefited or harmed, depending on the length of exposure.

Uses. Solar radiation toughens and thickens the skin, initiates the production of vitamin D, kills bacteria, modifies the activity of certain endocrine glands, and warms and relaxes the muscles. It also aids in the treatment of many nonpulmonary forms of tuberculosis.

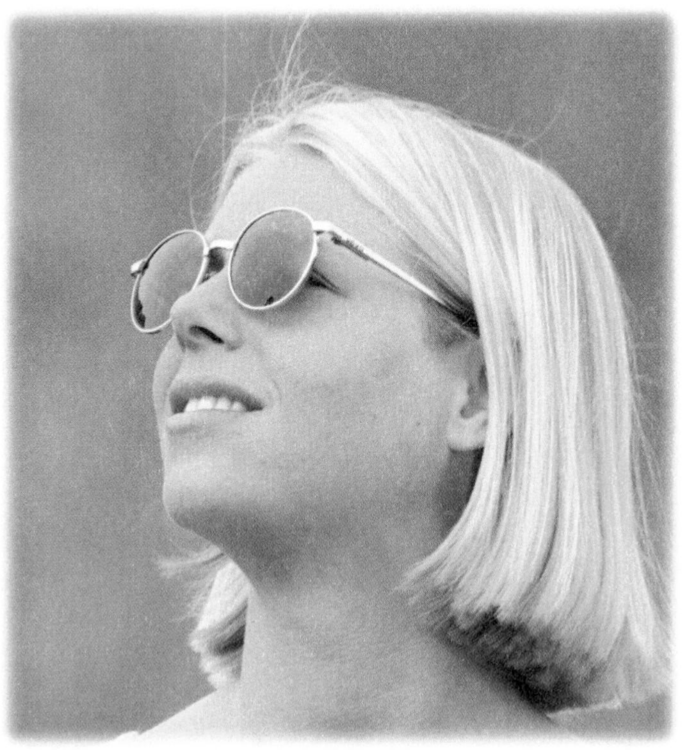

Contraindications. Avoid sun baths in cases of pulmonary tuberculosis and certain drugs that photosensitize the skin. If you are taking medications, check with your physician before taking a sun bath.

Procedure. In general, the sun bath is best taken before nine o'clock in the morning and after three o'clock in the afternoon. First expose a limited part of your skin for five minutes to direct sunlight and observe the next day if any burning has occurred. If you were sunburned, decrease the time of exposure; if not, increase the area exposed and the duration of exposure by one minute each day, exposing first the front of the body and then the back for the same length of time. It is unnecessary to expose the head, and the eyes should be shielded from direct exposure. Patients should be guarded from chilling, overheating, and overexposure.

It has been shown that fifteen minutes of daily exposure to the sun three times a week will provide all the vitamin D required by the body. Unfortunately, the same wavelengths that activate the production of vitamin D also cause aging of the skin and skin cancer. For this reason, a sunscreen (suntan lotion—available in drugstores) should be applied if longer and more frequent exposure is desired. However, it should be noted that sunscreens may effectively block the ultraviolet rays from penetrating the skin.

Dark-skinned persons require, on the average, six times the exposure to obtain the same physiological benefit as do light-skinned people. Blond, blue-eyed, and very fair-skinned people are the most susceptible to the sun's effects.

Sunlamps (ultraviolet lamps)

If it is not feasible to give a patient sun baths, but the effects of sun baths are desired, sunlamps, which provide the light spectrum desired, are available from *reliable* medical supply companies. The directions for their use should be followed carefully. Beware of the pseudoscientific claims made for various lamps on the market. Check with a physical therapist before making your purchase.

The uses, contraindications, and procedure for use are otherwise similar to those described under "sun baths." While sunlight is essential for life, avoid overexposure.

Massage

Massage is a system of remedial or hygienic manipulations of the body tissues with the hand or some instrument. It consists of rubbing, stroking, kneading, vibrating, or tapping. Although it is natural for a person to rub a part that may feel uncomfortable, the procedures of massage for the treatment of disease or injury are too complicated for a person to administer unless he has had proper training in an accredited institution. Massage by a well-trained therapist should be given only with the consent of a physician, and limited to the patient's specific needs.

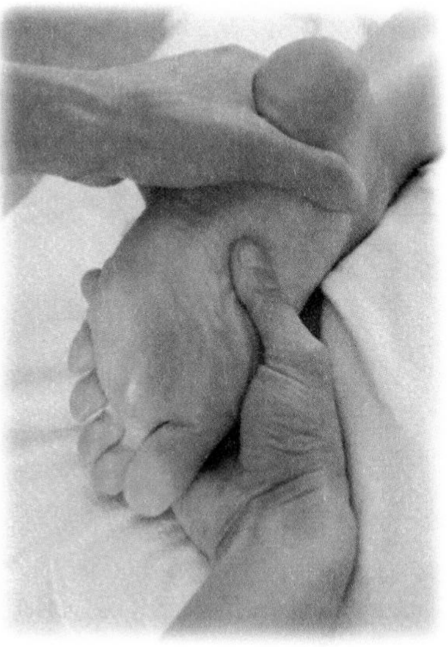

Massage by a well-trained therapist should be given only with the consent of a physician, and limited to the patient's specific needs.

It has been shown that fifteen minutes of daily exposure to the sun three times a week will provide all the vitamin D required by the body.

Progressive relaxation

Here is a simple way you can learn to relax overly tense muscles. Each learning session should last about twenty minutes. One or two sessions a day are sufficient.

Step 1. Lie on your back on a firm mattress or carpeted floor with your arms resting along your sides. Try to be as comfortable as possible.

Step 2. Relax your right hand at the wrist if you are right-handed, or your left hand if you are left-handed. This may take some time to learn. Some find that clenching the fist allows them to "feel" the muscles relax. When you think you have mastered this procedure, have a friend pick up your relaxed hand by a finger and let it go. If it fails to flop down, you are not ready to go on to the next step.

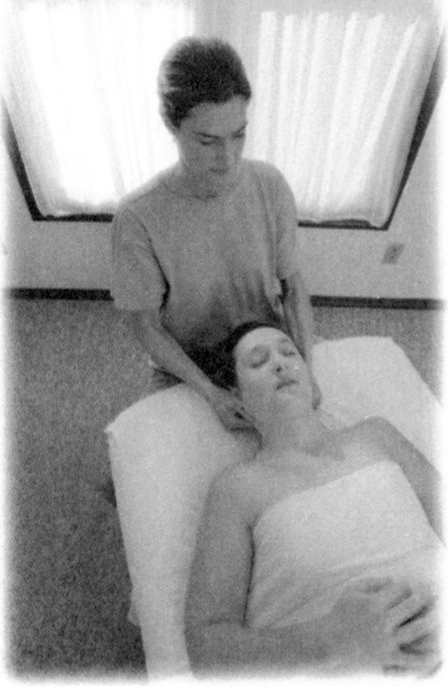

Step 3. Now relax your hand at the wrist and your forearm at the elbow. At each step, check to be sure you are really relaxed. Don't rush. It may take you several days to achieve the first step or two. Once you have mastered these, the others will come more rapidly.

Step 4. Now relax your hand at the wrist, your forearm at the elbow, and your arm at the shoulder. This will relax an entire upper limb.

Step 5. When you have accomplished the above, start on the opposite limb-hand at the wrist, forearm at the elbow, and arm at the shoulder. At the end of each session, relax both limbs together.

Step 6. Start on one of your lower limbs—the foot at the ankle, the leg at the knee, and the thigh at the hip, then the full lower limb. Now relax both upper limbs and the lower limb.

Step 7. Now do the other lower limb in the same step-by-step manner, relaxing all four limbs.

Step 8. Next concentrate on relaxing the muscles of your back. Follow this by relaxing the muscles of your abdomen and chest.

Step 9. Then relax the muscles of your neck so that your head is completely relaxed at the neck and shoulders.

Step 10. The final groups of muscles to relax are those of the face, scalp, and lower jaw (mandible). You should now be able to relax your entire body.

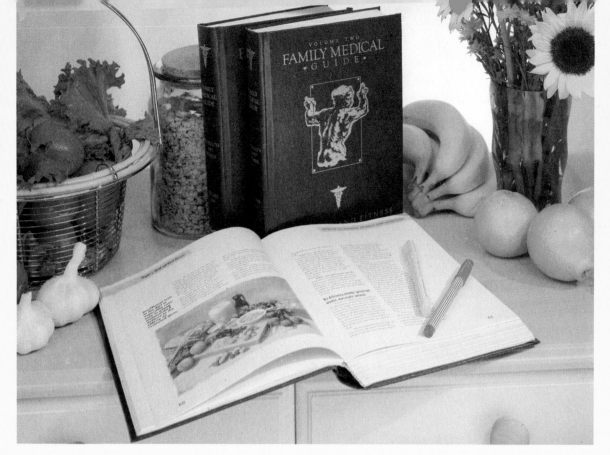

Great Stories for Kids

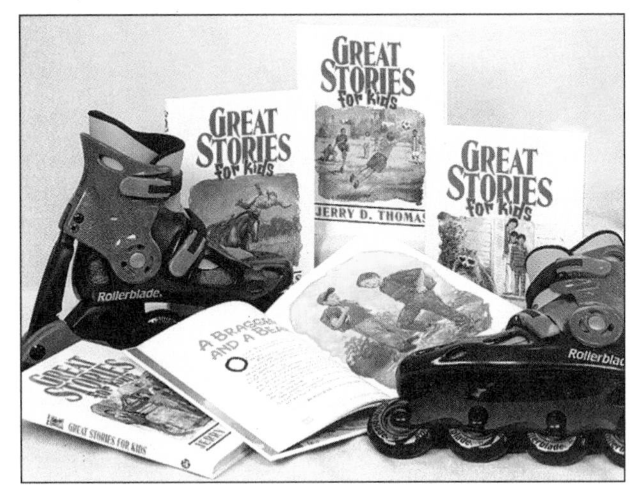

Your children will love the adventures and drama of the five-volume set *Great Stories for Kids,* and you'll value the character-building lessons they learn while reading these treasured stories. Each volume is bound in durable hardcover with delightful color illustrations. Also available in Spanish and French.

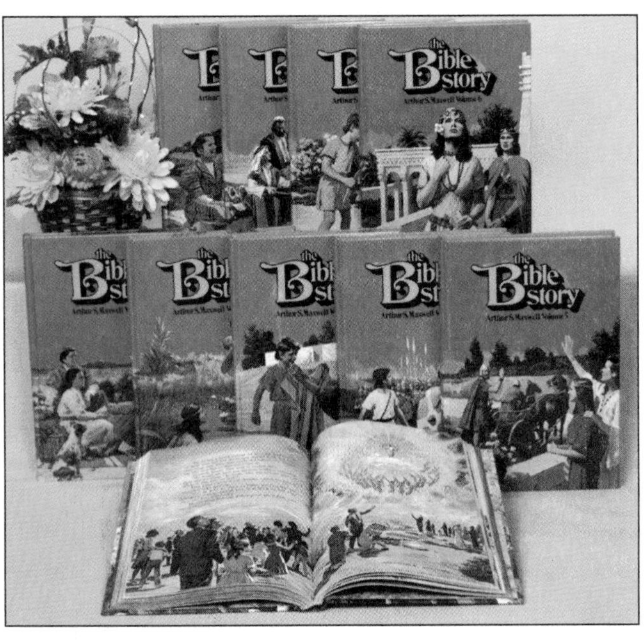

The Bible Story

The Bible Story was written not just to tell the wonderful stories in the Bible, but each story was especially written to teach your child a different character-building lesson—lessons such as honesty, respect for parents, obedience, kindness, and many more. This is truly the pleasant way to influence your child's character. The set contains more than 400 stories spread over 10 volumes. Hardcover.

Peace Above the Storm

People everywhere are searching for peace. They need power to cope with the "storms" in their lives. ***Peace Above the Storm*** is the answer to the problems people are facing today. This all-time bestseller; printed in more than 100 languages, has already brought comfort and inspiration to millions of readers. Topics such as "Freedom From Guilt," "Discovering Peace of Mind," "Becoming a New Person," "The Power of Prayer," "Unconditional Love," and others could make this the most important book you have ever read.

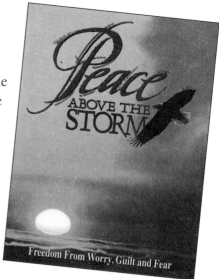

For more information, mail the postpaid card, or write to:
Pacific Press Marketing Service, P.O. Box 5353, Nampa, ID 83653.

Yes, please send me information on the following:

- ❑ FAMILY MEDICAL GUIDE TO HEALTH AND FITNESS
- ❑ GREAT STORIES FOR KIDS
- ❑ THE BIBLE STORY
- ❑ PEACE ABOVE THE STORM

Name______________________________

Address____________________________

City_______________________________

State________Zip_______________

Phone (   )______________________

STUDY THE BIBLE BY MAIL

The free Discover Bible study guides help you find The answers to life's most important questions.

- SUFFERING—Why does God permit it? Does God really care?
- LIFE AFTER DEATH—What will it be like?
- PRAYER—How can I know God will hear and answer me?

Get your first lesson by returning this card with your name and address.

Name______________________________

Street______________ Apt. ________

City_______________________________

State______ Zip _______________

BUSINESS REPLY MAIL
FIRST-CLASS MAIL PERMIT NO. 300 NAMPA ID

POSTAGE WILL BE PAID BY ADDRESSEE

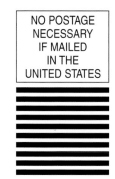

PACIFIC PRESS® PUBLISHING ASSOCIATION
MARKETING SERVICE
PO BOX 5353
NAMPA ID 83653-9903

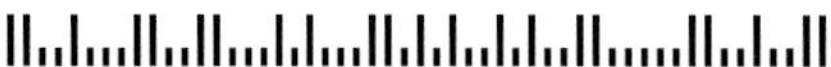

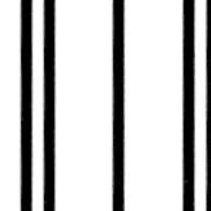

PLACE
STAMP
HERE

DISCOVER
PO BOX 53055
LOS ANGELES CA 90053-0055